MEDICAL JOURNALS AND MEDICAL KNOWLEDGE

THE WELLCOME INSTITUTE SERIES IN THE HISTORY OF MEDICINE

Edited by W.F. Bynum and Roy Porter,
The Wellcome Institute

Medical Fringe and Medical Orthodoxy, 1750–1850
W.F. Bynum and Roy Porter
Florence Nightingale and the Nursing Legacy
Monica Baly
Social Hygiene in Twentieth Century Britain
Greta Jones
Problems and Methods in the History of Medicine
Roy Porter and Andrew Wear
Vivisection in Historical Perspective
Nicolaas A. Rupke
(Now available in paperback)
Abortion in England, 1919–1967
Barbara Brookes
The Hospital in History
Lindsay Granshaw and Roy Porter
(Now available in paperback)
Women as Mothers in Pre-Industrial England
Valerie Fildes
Birth Control in Germany, 1871–1933
James Woycke
The Charitable Imperative
Colin Jones
Medicine at the Courts of Europe, 1500–1837
Vivian Nutton
Mad Tales from the Raj
Waltraud Ernst
British Medicine in an Age of Reform
Roger French and Andrew Wear
Doctor of Society
Roy Porter

MEDICAL JOURNALS AND MEDICAL KNOWLEDGE

HISTORICAL ESSAYS

Edited by
W.F. Bynum, Stephen Lock and Roy Porter

ROUTLEDGE

London and New York

First published in 1992
by Routledge
11 New Fetter Lane, London EC4P 4EE

Simultaneously published in the USA and Canada
by Routledge
a division of Routledge, Chapman and Hall Inc.
29 West 35th Street, New York, NY 10001

Typeset by LaserScript, Mitcham, Surrey
Printed and bound in Great Britain by
Biddles Ltd, Guildford and King's Lynn

British Library Cataloguing in Publication Data
Medical journals and medical knowledge: historical essays.
1. Medicine. History
I. Bynum, W.F. (William Frederick) *1943–* II. Lock,
Stephen III. Porter, Roy *1946–* IV. Series
610.9

Library of Congress Cataloging in Publication Data
Medical journals and medical knowledge: historical essays/edited by
W.F. Bynum, Stephen Lock, and Roy Porter.
p. cm. – (The Wellcome Institute series in the history of medicine)
Includes bibliographical references and index.
1. Journalism, Medical – United States – History – 18th century.
2. Medical writing – Periodicals – United States – History.
3. Communication in medicine – United States – History. 4. Medical
literature – United States – History. I. Bynum, W.F. (William F.),
1943– . II. Lock, Stephen. III. Porter, Roy, 1946– .
IV. Series.
[DNLM: 1. Periodicals – history – essays. 2. Publishing – history –
essays. WZ 345 M4885]
PN4784.M4M38 1992
070.4′4961 – dc20
DNLM/DLC
for Library of Congress 91–25779
CIP

ISBN 0–415–07025–2

Contents

Figures and tables

Figures

Tables

Contributors

Peter Bartrip is a research associate in social history at the Centre for Socio-Legal Studies at Wolfson College, Oxford. He is currently writing a commissioned history of the British Medical Association.

Sir Christopher Booth was professor of medicine at the Royal Postgraduate Medical School, and subsequently director of the Clinical Research Centre, Northwick Park. He is now Harveian Librarian of the Royal College of Physicians.

William H. Brock is reader in the history of science at the University of Leicester. He has published extensively on the history of chemistry, the history of science education and the development of science periodicals. Books include *Atomic Debates* (1967), *H.E. Armstrong and the Teaching of Science* (1973), *The Lamp of Learning* (with A.J. Meadows, 1984) and *From Protyle to Proton* (1985).

John C. Burnham is professor of history at the Ohio State University. His publications are chiefly in the fields of the history of psychiatry, the history of the medical profession, and the social and intellectual history of American science and culture.

W.F. Bynum is head of the Academic Unit at the Wellcome Institute for the History of Medicine, and reader in the history of medicine at University College London. He has published widely on many aspects of the history of the biomedical and life sciences and, with Roy Porter, is general editor of the Wellcome Institute Series in the History of Medicine.

Michael Harris lectures in history at the Centre for Extramural Studies at Birkbeck College. He has edited a series of volumes on the history of the book trade, is author of *London Newspapers in the Age of Walpole* and has written extensively on the development of the print culture. He is general editor of the *Journal of Newspaper and Periodical History*.

Elizabeth Knoll is an acquiring editor for science and history of science at the University of California Press and a former member of staff of the *Journal of the American Medical Association*. She wrote a Ph.D. in the history of evolutionary ideas at the University of Chicago and has written on editorial peer review and scientific publications.

Jane Lewis is a reader in social administration at the London School of Economics and Political Science. She is the author of several books and articles on women's history, as well as a study of informal care (with Barbara Meredith), *Daughters who Care* (1988), and a history of the philosophy and practice of public health, *What Price Community Medicine?* (1986).

Stephen Lock was the Editor of the *British Medical Journal* from 1975 to 1991 and is now a free-lance journalist and medical historian. Among his many books is *A Difficult Balance* (1985), a study of the peer review system in medicine.

Jean Loudon is compiling an index of obituaries of medical practitioners appearing in medical journals from 1750 to 1850.

Irvine Loudon is a medical historian. His *Medical Care and the General Practitioner, 1750–1850* (Oxford University Press) was published in 1986. He is currently completing an international study of maternal care and maternal mortality from 1800 to 1950.

Roy Porter is senior lecturer in the social history of medicine at the Wellcome Institute for the History of Medicine. Recent books include *Patient's Progress* (co-authored with Dorothy Porter, 1989), *Health For Sale: Quackery in England, 1660–1850* (1990) and *Doctor of Society: Thomas Beddoes and the Sick Trade in Late-enlightenment England* (1991).

Ruth Richardson works on the Builder Project at the Institute of Historical Research, University of London. Her book *Death, Dissection and the Destitute* was published in 1988.

Michael Shepherd is emeritus professor of epidemiological psychiatry at the Institute of Psychiatry, University of London.

Julian Tudor Hart was a general practitioner for five years in London, and for 27 years in South Wales. He is now on the scientific staff of the Medical Research Council's Epidemiology and Medical Care Unit, and is lecturer in the Department of General Practice at St Mary's Hospital Medical School. His book, *A New Kind of Doctor* (1988), is a social history of British general practice in the twentieth century.

Janice Wilson is a librarian in the reader services department at the Wellcome Institute for the History of Medicine, London.

Acknowledgements

This volume has arisen out of a conference held at the Royal Institution in September 1990 to mark the 150th anniversary of the founding of the *British Medical Journal*. The editors would like to extend thanks to all who helped with funding and organizing that conference; and to all those attenders whose participation contributed so much to make the ensuing discussions exceptionally lively. The papers here published have benefited greatly.

It is sad to have to record that two speakers invited to participate died before the conference took place: Edward Kass and Eli Chernin. Dr. Chernin's paper, 'An informal tour of the early British and American journals of tropical medicine and hygiene', will appear in *Medical History*, 36 (1), January 1992.

Invaluable secretarial help with this volume has been given by Gaby Shockley, Frieda Houser and Sally Bragg. The index has been compiled, immaculately as ever, by Jean Runciman.

Introduction

The history of medical journalism has largely been ignored; yet who can deny its immense impact?

In the seventeenth-century 'Battle of the Books' over the comparative virtues of Classical and Modern learning, defenders of the Moderns typically claimed that the key to their superiority over the Ancients lay in the invention of printing. The Gutenberg age, claimed Modernists from Bacon to Voltaire and the *philosophes*, had guaranteed for the first time the easy, inexpensive and exact preservation and diffusion of knowledge; in fact, the reproductive technology of the printing press had rendered information a force in the public domain which, despite all the endeavours of censors, had for ever slipped the reins of rigid central control. This was doubtless a propaganda claim, but recent historians of print culture, notably Elizabeth Eisenstein,[1] have emphasized that it also contained a core of truth. It is now commonly argued by historians of science that the transformation of attitudes towards Nature that we call the Scientific Revolution owed as much to the new styles of thinking required by the printed scientific paper as to the pioneering of experimentation and the invention of the laboratory.[2] And print made a particularly powerful impact upon the spread and advance of medical knowledge, because of the crucial importance to medical instruction of the reproducibility of standardized, stereotyped anatomical and physiological illustrations, made possible by the techniques of woodcutting, engraving and, finally, photography.[3]

Nevertheless books clearly existed before printing; or, in other words, the advent of printing did not so much create the book as globalize it. A stronger claim may be made for the journal. Before Gutenberg, it may make no sense at all to speak of medico-scientific journals. Of course, news of developments in these fields of enquiry travelled in written form, as well as by word of mouth, before the Renaissance, but such communication was essentially individual and private, through letters and the like. It was printing that made possible that special engine of data-recording and sounding-board of opinion which established itself from the mid-seventeenth century as the medico-scientific journal, and effected a qualitative transformation in knowledge in the process.

Considering their vast importance, past and present, it is remarkable that the history of scientific, technical and medical journals has been so little studied. There is no substantial modern study even of the *Philosophical Transactions of the Royal Society*, no book-length history of *Nature*. And the same applies to the field of medicine. Although, as the notes to the present volume indicate, the field has not been wholly neglected – and, of course, a history of the *British Medical Journal* has recently appeared[4] – it is remarkable that we know so little about the roots of medical journalism, about the development of the typical form and format of the journal, about editorial practices, about the finances of the medical press, and about the precise ways in which medical journalism altered the world of medicine proper.

Remarkable, but not impossible to explain. For one thing, it has been very easy in Britain to engage in a chain of reasoning which assumes that medical journalism 'began' (really or virtually) with *The Lancet*, indeed is somehow epitomized by *The Lancet*, and that the history of *The Lancet* is in turn itself encapsulated in the attitudes and activities of its first editor, Thomas Wakley. Hence, by a historical sleight of hand, the history of British medical journalism becomes dissolved into the career of Thomas Wakley.[5] The present volume does not come to bury Wakley: far from it; and various of the contributors discuss his significance. But it is important to recognize that the importance of *The Lancet* rested not in laying the foundation stone of British medical journalism, but, in some measure, in challenging its norms and changing its directions; and that many other journals of the first half of the nineteenth century were also influential within medicine and pioneering within the general field of technical publishing. The essays in the first half of the volume – by Roy Porter, W.F. Bynum and Janice Wilson, William

Brock, and Irvine and Jean Loudon – all establish the contexts and contents of medical journalism up to the mid-Victorian age.

There is a further reason for neglect. By training and inclination, historians are generally more interested in content than in form. Tracing discoveries, analysing ideas, establishing priorities, laying controversies bare, plotting influences, finding hidden meanings: these are the central activities of medical historians. They are interested in the words on the page, rather than the page itself, and the place of the page within the wider media of information dispersal and preservation. The result can often be a kind of blindness, compounded by present-mindedness. We are so used to living in a world of instantaneous, near-infallible information dissemination that it is sometimes difficult to think ourselves back into the communications milieux of a couple of centuries ago, in which 'discoveries' could all too easily remain undiscovered for years or even generations, simply because the material media of communications – print, the postal services, library facilities, and so forth – were so defective. Or, to put this another way, we of the journal-era – and beyond – have to make a special leap of imagination to grasp the difference made by the advent of the journal. Hence, one of the questions addressed by many of the contributions below – and of course remaining for further researchers – is the difference to the economy of medical knowledge made by the coming of regular repositories of news, information and opinion. How much more certain, how much more speedy, did data dissemination become? What impact did this have upon the making of the medical community itself? Clearly, the medical journal recorded and reflected medical change (as Sir Christopher Booth very elegantly demonstrates below): how far did it also serve as an engine actually for *shaping* the future of medicine?

Certain themes assume repeated prominence in the discussions below. Several essays seek to place medical journals and medical issues within the wider world of the press and public opinion. Michael Harris examines the standing of doctors and the writing of medical 'scandal' within the popular press of mid-Victorian England, indirectly revealing precisely why the professional medical press proper was at such pains to establish its own credentials and respectability. William Brock examines the interplay between the domains of medical and scientific writing; Michael Shepherd looks at the rise of a specialized psychiatric press; while Ruth Richardson surveys another branch of Victorian journalism – the architectural press – likewise with a view to establishing the 'spillage' from one field to another. Are we dealing in the mid-Victorian age with a public composed of supposedly omniscient and omnivorous general readers, who take all learning as their parish? Or do we see incipient specialization? Jane Lewis's discussion of the reporting of public health issues would certainly suggest that, as the medical profession itself grew more specialized, a division of labour, and even of sympathies, emerged alongside within medical press publishing.

Whereas, as Peter Bartrip emphasizes in his discussion of the crusading activities of the greatest Victorian editor of the *British Medical Journal*, Ernest Hart, the *BMJ* in its early years could act as a general campaigning paper, for much of the twentieth century it developed the tendency to look in upon itself, and devote itself to essentially internal concerns (professional organization, medical research). Yet to make this point is not to imply some 'natural law' of increased specialization. For, as Julian Tudor Hart is at pains to argue, journals (especially official professional-association organs) also act as ideological mouthpieces reflecting the changing political orientations of readers/members – a point repeatedly addressed in Elizabeth Knoll's parallel study of *JAMA*.

The essays in this volume directly and implicitly raise big issues. Many of these cannot as yet be answered, for want of the requisite information at our fingertips: aggregate circulation figures, details of the mechanics of the editorial process, of refereeing practices, and so forth, and, not least, hard evidence of how and how far the journals which were produced were actually read – and by whom? The following pages, however, do fill in many of the gaps in our knowledge of these matters. John Burnham's meticulous citation-study charts the changing fortunes of the *British Medical Journal* in North America, and thereby opens up a range of fascinating questions about reciprocities in Anglo–American medical exchange over the last century.

In the development of the scholarly division of labour, medical historians have developed their own 'separate sphere', distinct from historians of the press, publishing and periodicals. What this volume abundantly shows are the pitfalls of such arbitrary separations of the medium from the message. Reflecting upon the history of the medical journal reminds us that it is at our peril that we divide knowledge from its technological, material and economic bases.

Notes

1. E. Eisenstein (1979) *The Printing Press as an Agent of Change*, 2 vols, Cambridge: Cambridge University Press.

2. J.V. Golinski, 'Language, Discourse and Science', in R.C. Olby, G.N. Cantor, J.R.R. Christie, and M.J.S. Hodge (eds), *Companion to the History of Modern Science* (London: Routledge, 1990), 110–26. For contemporary theories of language, see Hans Aarsleff, *From Locke to Saussure: Essays on the Study of Language and Intellectual History* (Minneapolis, Minn.: University of Minnesota Press, 1982); Brian Vickers and Nancy S. Struever, *Rhetoric and the Pursuit of Truth: Language Change in the Seventeenth and Eighteenth Centuries: Papers read at a Clark Library Seminar 8 March 1980* (Los Angeles, Calif.: William Andrews Clark Memorial Library, University of California, Los Angeles, 1985); Walter J. Ong (1979) *Interfaces of the Word: Studies in the Evolution of Consciousness and Culture*, Ithaca: Cornell University Press; *idem* (1982) *Orality and Literacy: The Technologizing of the Word*, London: Methuen; *idem* (1967) *The Presence of the Word: Some Prolegomena for Cultural and Religious History*, New Haven: Yale University Press. For experiment and the laboratory see Simon Schaffer and Steven Shapin (1984) *Leviathan and the Air Pump*, Princeton: Princeton University Press; Bruno Latour (1988) *The Pasteurization of France*, Cambridge, Mass.: Harvard University Press.

3. John L. Thornton (1966) *Medical Books, Libraries and Collectors: A Study of Bibliography and the Book Trade in Relation to the Medical Sciences*, 2nd ed., London: André Deutsch.

4. Peter Bartrip (1990) *Mirror of Medicine. A History of the BMJ*, Oxford: Oxford University Press.

5. S.S. Sprigge (1897) *The Life and Times of Thomas Wakley*, London: Longmans & Co.

1

The rise of medical journalism in Britain to 1800

Roy Porter

We seem to be drowning in print. 'Like beach plums', grumbles Gerald Weissmann, 'new journals appear in crops overnight. . . . There are too many of them, they are published too often, they stare from the racks and reproach us for sloth'.[1]

Were things different in the past? Instructing a young physician in his duties, the Revd Thomas Gisborne urged him to keep up. 'The Medical Journals of eminence published in foreign countries, as well as those established in his own, will properly engage his attention. From the one and the other he will probably derive very important assistance in the discharge of his duty as a Physician'.[2] The youngster might even wish to contribute, though, here as elsewhere, the evangelical Gisborne warned of vainglory:[3]

> He will not subject himself, by committing his thoughts to the press without sufficient previous enquiry, to the charge of purloining the discoveries of others; nor of being vain of communicating what is either unworthy of notice, or as yet but feebly and imperfectly developed, or hastily inferred from few and inadequate trials.

Gisborne fretted over the poisonous passions of print, warning the novice that 'if, through any thing which he has done, or of any thing which he has published, he should find himself driven into a controversy' he must 'conduct the literary warfare with becoming temper'.[4] The date? 1794. Clearly, the delights and dangers of the medical journal were well known by the close of the eighteenth century.

The centuries after Gutenberg naturally saw a proliferation of medical publishing: monographs, syllabuses, pamphlets, quacks' handbills, textbooks and anatomy atlases, targeted at professionals, students and even the public.[5] In the seventeenth century there were, in practice, no exclusively medical journals anywhere. Medical matters were, however, aired in the new scientific journals sprouting from mid-century: in Britain, in the *Philosophical Transactions* of the Royal Society; in France, in the *Journal des Scavans* of the Académie Royale des Sciences; in the Germanies, the *Acta Eruditorum* (1682).[6] Historians often convey the impression that astronomy and physics were at the heart of the scientific revolution. Maybe, but quantitatively what filled the meetings of scientific societies and the pages of their publications were natural history, botany, zoology, anatomy, physiology and all aspects of medicine, theoretical, experimental, clinical and pathological. Open *Phil. Trans.* for 1667 and you immediately light upon a medical event of great significance: 'An Account of More Tryals of Transfusion . . . The Method of Transfusing into the Veines of Men'.[7] The prominence of medicine should come as no surprise: physicians like Martin Lister, Hans Sloane and James Jurin were amongst the Royal Society's most active officers.[8]

The quantity of medical material in general scientific journals diminished during the eighteenth century. Doctors continued, of course, to avail themselves of traditional publishing outlets: handsome volumes, such as William Hunter's *The Human Gravid Uterus*, went on sale alongside the vitriol of medical pamphlet wars in the golden age of Grub Street.[9] And they exploited new publishing openings; to a small degree, the newspaper (mainly colonized by quacks),[10] but mainly the superior monthly periodicals catering for polite and enlightened readerships. John Fothergill, John Coakley Lettsom, and many another élite practitioner sent their items to the *Gentleman's Magazine*, a general-interest periodical with a circulation touching 10,000, which regularly carried essays on disease prevention, drugs, first aid, epidemics, and the new charity hospitals, as well as offering reviews of medical books, a battleground for professional altercations and a forum for what was termed a 'medical correspondence'. Contributors to the *Gent's Mag.* argued for closer communications between public and profession, urging jargon-free writing and easy information exchange.[11]

But this was the time that also saw the specialist medical serial emerge.[12] 'Hunt the first medical journal' is a rather arid parlour game: scores of medical publications came out, promising a regular appearance, only to disappear before anyone even noticed them. Some of the earliest were ephemeral indeed. After the brief glory in 1682 of the *Weekly Memorials for the Ingenious*, which carried abstracts and reviews, many of them medical, *Medicina Curiosa* appeared on 17 June 1684, claiming to offer 'a variety of new communications in physick, chirurgery and anatomy', but never got beyond its second issue in October: about par for the course for early serials.[13]

The eighteenth century saw more durable productions. Here the pioneers were handsome collections of substantial papers, brought out occasionally under the direction of bodies of medical gentlemen: the *Medical Essays and Observations*, produced by a society in Edinburgh, which appeared in six volumes between 1733 and 1744; its successor, the *Essays and Observations*, published in Edinburgh in three volumes between 1754 and 1765; the *Medical Observations and Inquiries*, issued by a 'Society of Physicians' in London, which appeared erratically in six volumes between 1757 and 1784; the *Medical Transactions*, published in six tomes by the Royal College of Physicians of London from 1768 to 1820. The *Memoirs of the Medical Society of London* first appeared in 1787, continuing under than name, through six volumes, till 1805;[14] and so forth. More specialized groups also pressed into print: the Royal Humane Society published its *Reports* from 1775 to 1795[15] and, thanks to the energetic John Haygarth, the Chester Society for Promoting Inoculation its own *Proceedings* from 1778 to 1782.

In time, something more closely resembling a regular commercial medical press established itself. The *Medical Museum*, claiming on its title page to be 'a repository of cases, experiments, researches and discoveries, collected at home and abroad', came out monthly in two annual volumes, and reached a third volume before going under in 1764. The *Foreign Medical Review* appeared in four parts in two volumes between 1779 and 1780 before folding. The *London Medical Journal* was founded by Dr Samuel Foart Simmons in 1781; ten years later, it changed its name, presumably to gain a splash of novelty, to *Medical Facts and Observations*, and lasted till 1800. The *Medical Spectator* managed forty-eight ordinary and two extraordinary numbers between 1791 and 1796; the *Medical and Chirurgical Review* appeared in sixteen regular volumes between 1794 and 1808: the *Annals of Medicine* started in 1796, going on under that masthead till 1804, when it was born again as the *Edinburgh Medical and Surgical Journal* of distinguished reputation. Around 1800, there sprang up the *London Medical Review and Magazine*, and the *Medical and Physical Journal*.

By now, we have gained familiar ground. A quite extensive medical press was operating by 1800 – over thirty titles had come and gone; and if few journals achieved any longevity before collapsing, or being renamed, new ones were always plugging the gaps. A formula was emerging – a core of cases and clinical materials, spiced with some news, copious book reviewing and a dash of correspondence, which makes them recognizable precursors of *The Lancet* or the *BMJ*. Not least, in 1799, a prospectus appeared for a monthly *British Medical Journal* itself. If it ever appeared, no copy seems to survive.[16]

Thus: the birth of British medical journals. There is no room here to examine their contents in any detail. But it is worth posing some broader questions: why did medical journalism emerge when it did? Why did it assume its particular form? What problems, what prospects, did it create for medical knowledge? Pre-modern medicine was beset by formidable difficulties regarding its public face, professional organization, ethical codes and scientific authority. However halting and uneven, the development of medical journalism in an Enlightenment age preoccupied with questions of knowledge, truth and power may be seen as a response to these challenges.[17]

Crucial was the question of information: its status, its proprietorship. Should medical knowledge be free and open? Or were there occasions for secrecy? Were some, but only some, chambers of the medical mansion fit for public viewing? Should knowledge have its private parts?[18]

If medicine was to be seen to be a progressive body of scientific knowledge, surely (many argued) it had to fulfil the Baconian criterion of being freely communicated and fairly criticized: 'communications must run through all ye veines of ye Main worke', John Beale had assured Henry Oldenburg, secretary to the Royal Society, in 1662.[19] But there were carping voices claiming that, in actuality, medicine was the reverse, a closed shop, resting on hidebound authorities. Appalled at the stagnation of medical science, the late eighteenth-century reformer, Dr Thomas Beddoes, blamed the want of effective machinery for the storage and circulation of information. The protocols of private and medical practice discouraged data-pooling.[20]

To all responsible opinion, barefaced secretiveness in a mortal matter such as clinical medicine (most notoriously, concealment of the composition of medicaments) was an abomination. 'Secrecy, as you well know, and promises unrestrained by sense of shame', Beddoes assured his colleague, Erasmus Darwin, 'constitute the *essential character* of empiricism'.[21] Little less harmful, however, Beddoes judged, was the near-universal oblivion which overtook clinical know-how. Mountains of valuable data were being daily registered in the brains, and even the notebooks, of doctors: what a scandal that most vanished without trace.[22] Such 'waste of facts' was shocking, for 'the grand expedient for rendering physiology popular and medicine certain, is to enlarge our stock of observations on animal nature'.[23]

Beddoes proposed two solutions. First, systematic collection and indexing of medical facts.[24] 'Why should not reports be transmitted at fixed periods from all the hospitals and medical charities in the kingdom to a central board?'[25] Other 'charitable establishments for the relief of the indigent sick' must also supply information, as should physicians at large.[26] Data should be processed by a paid clerical staff, and made freely available. Seminars should be held. The stimulus to comparison and criticisms would sift good practice from bad. 'What would be the effect', Beddoes mused, of 'register offices, not exactly for receiving votive tablets, like certain ancient temples, but in which attestations, both of the good and of the evil, that appears to be done by practitioners of medicine, should be deposited?'[27] Without effective information storage, retrieval and dissemination, medicine would never take its place amongst the progressive sciences.[28] 'To lose a single fact may be to lose many lives. Yet ten thousand, perhaps, are lost for one that is preserved; and all for want of a system among our theatres of disease, combined with the establishment of a national bank of medical wealth, where each individual practitioner may deposit his gains of knowledge, and draw out, in return, the stock, accumulated by all his brethren'.[29]

Second, to complement his medical bank, Beddoes urged his fellows to publish more. He was himself a tireless author – some thirty books, a score of articles and hundreds of book reviews; he himself edited *Contributions to Physical and Medical Knowledge*

(1799),[30] a compendium of papers written largely by his friends. Not least, he contributed to such new organs as the *Medical and Physical Journal* and *Medical Facts and Information*. Looking back, he argued it was no accident that Vesalius had followed hard on Gutenberg's heels, thereby ensuring the superiority of the medical Moderns over the Ancients.[31]

Greater diffusion of knowledge, better medicine: an attractive formula. But there were counter-arguments. Was not the cornerstone of medicine the bedside encounter? And crucial to this, surely, was the contract of confidentiality. Would it not be improper to broadcast case histories, involving necessarily intimate details about identifiable patients?[32]

Thus medicine – though not, say, chemistry – was beset by competing imperatives. For progress, knowledge had to be published. But bedside etiquette required privacy, above all in delicate areas such as mental illness or obstetrics.[33]

And assuming knowledge ought to be publicized, what were the proper channels? Was all medical knowledge fit for public consumption? Or should certain sorts of information be on restricted access, for professional eyes alone? These issues flared in two controversial areas.

First, conflicts between orthodox doctors and empirics.[34] Regulars accused quacks of dastardly secrecy, above all respecting their nostrums. Quacks retorted that it was the regulars who hid knowledge from the public behind the closed doors of such secret societies as the College of Physicians, veiled in dead languages and arcane terminologies.[35] And quacks astutely counter-appealed to the public as the tribunal of truth. This was a tricky ploy to meet, as Lettsom discovered in the 1770s when he tried to scotch the uroscopist, Theodor Myersbach. Lettsom tilted against the German in the newspapers, but, while soliciting public support, he also accused newspaper readers of stupidity in patronizing quacks, and insisted that doctors knew best. Appealing to a public, of whom he was contemptuous to their faces, Lettsom was hoist on his own petard.[36]

But larger issues were at stake than this row between a quack and a Quaker. In those days before modern scientific medicine, buttressed by the teaching hospital, the university department, the lab, the MRC and even, of course, the medical journal, who authorized medical truth? Wherein was it grounded? In musty tomes? In experiments? In the *ipse dixits* of scientists? In shows of hands, the shouts of the public, or the sick voting with their feet? Was medical knowledge meritocratic, aristocratic or democratic?

The conundrums of public knowledge[37] surfaced in other ways. Was the publishing doctor a public benefactor? Or was he a self-serving self-publicist? Many felt obliged to defend themselves on this score. 'Public utility, and not a mere *scabies scribendi*', argued Dr Cook, not wholly convincingly, in the *Gentleman's Magazine*, 'is the only motive of my writing so often'.[38] And this raised a further issue: how far should the public be *au fait* with medicine, with a view to self-help and informed decision-making? Many regular, but radical, doctors, notably William Buchan, believed it was high time to lay medicine bare. There was little in the medical art beyond the talents of a well-informed layman. Through his best-selling *Domestic Medicine*, Buchan sought to make everyone, in all but name, his own physician.[39]

Other doctors saw red. Polite society, pinning misplaced faith on its own medical know-how, and assuming that payers of pipers should call the tunes, already interfered far too much, retorted Beddoes, to medicine's disgrace and the ruin of their constitutions. Great evils resulted from the public poring over 'home doctor' texts.[40] Assuredly knowledge must be broadcast more energetically, but to practitioners not the public.

But how could 'restricted circulation' be justified by progressives – as Beddoes saw himself – in the age of the Enlightenment?[41] Freedom of information was an Enlightenment shibboleth: monopoly and censorship contravened the spirit of an age urging free markets in knowledge no less than in loaves.

And this raises a final bone of contention: profit. On the one hand, publishing opened prospects of reward. In the eighteenth century, medicine followed market opportunities, bold as brass (the bilious Beddoes dubbed it 'the sick trade').[42] Publishing popular pamphlets and high-visibility books offered attractions for some physicians at least. They might make money, they might also make a name: and who was to draw the lines between responsible diffusion of information and arrant opportunism?[43]

Yet business sense dissuaded others from publishing at all. Many leading Scottish medical professors, as also the great William Hunter, London's top anatomy school proprietor, never printed their lectures, lest this jeopardize their lucrative lecturing income.[44] Thus it could be profitable not to rush into print. Yet, taken too far, such closeness with information itself risked becoming the 'secrecy' for which the nostrum-vending quack was reviled.[45]

And, in any case, there were countervailing pressures urging publication upon the likes of Hunter. These were not today's 'publish or perish' anxieties. But one had to authenticate one's originality, the exclusive rights to one's own literary products. Literary historians have contended that our modern concept of the author as exclusive begetter and proprietor of his own brainchildren is itself the product of print culture. Certainly copyright laws were passed during the eighteenth century, to provide some measure of legal protection against plagiarists and pirates. The medical journal could offer a speedy way to establish priority.[46]

In short, the relations in Georgian England between medical knowledge and medical publishing were not simple. After the lapsing of the Licensing Act in 1695, publishing was a booming business. But a medical world in which aspiring practitioners had to look more to lay patrons than to their peers for name and fame hardly provided the best seedbed for a specialist medical press. Contrast the far more favourable conditions obtaining in the Victorian age: a heightened sense of professional *esprit de corps* and exclusiveness, concentrated in clubs, societies and associations, disciplinary specialization, radical reform campaigns, and all those other features later conspicuous in the pages of *The Lancet* and the *BMJ*.[47]

Nevertheless, the Georgian century did see the origins of a medical press.[48] How, and how effectively, did it surmount the obstacles I have surveyed? It is time to plunge into the texts.

Amongst the more stable and successful, if staid, progeny of the Georgian medical press were the collections of papers put out by medical societies, such as the *Medical Observations and Inquiries*, the work of an *ad hoc* group of London physicians – mainly young, Scottish and thwarted – whose first volume appeared in 1757. Its preface observed tartly that it was some 'reflection on the faculty' that the College had not already launched into print. *Medical Observations and Inquiries* championed Baconian empiricism. 'Hypothetical disquisitions, points of controversy, numerous and needless quotations, in short, whatever has rather a tendency to show the parts and erudition of the writer, than to advance medical knowledge, will be suppressed.'[49] Aside from brief editorial comments – for instance self-congratulation over the progress of smallpox inoculation[50] – *Medical Observations and Inquiries* consisted wholly of clinical papers, generally substantial case histories by such major figures as John Fothergill, William Hunter, Gowin Knight and John Clephane.[51]

Eventually the College was stung into action, producing *Medical Transactions Published by the Royal College of Physicians in London* (1785). Medicine had been fast advancing since the seventeenth century, announced its pious prefatory platitudes, thanks to the founding of medical societies. This advance would now be accelerated by publication, or, in their pompous prose, 'as the art of physic hath been so much improved by this method of communicating observations, the College of Physicians in London are desirous of furthering a design so worthy of their attention'.[52]

Here the epistemological problem raised earlier – how publications could be avouched as authentic – was obviated by the fact that all the authors were members of the College – indeed, they included its doyens such as William Heberden – and their papers had previously been delivered before it. Publication was thus less an act than its record. Even so, a corporate disclaimer was judged prudent: 'The College think it proper to declare that they do not, as a body, mean to vouch for the truth of any relation, or to give authority to any opinion, contained in the papers here published'.[53]

The College's *Medical Transactions* has a certain sedate, inhouse air. Yet once an organ passes into the public domain, it takes on a life of its own. This is evident in what might otherwise seem a surprising contribution to the third volume, 'A Letter . . . Concerning the Angina Pectoris', 'introduced' by Heberden who noted: 'Soon after the publication of the second volume of the *Medical Transactions*, I received the following anonymous letter. "Sir, Seeing among the extracts of the *Medical Transactions* in the *Critical Review* of last month, your account of a disorder, which you term the *angina pectoris*, I find it so exactly correspond with what I have experienced of late years, that it determined me to give you such particulars"' – which the author then proceeded to enumerate, before Heberden made further observations of his own.[54] It is a telling instance. It shows what is called the 'bridging effect' – the diffusion of originally restricted and arcane material to wider audiences through the agency of popularizing media (the *Critical Review* was a general-interest monthly specializing in book-reviewing).[55] It shows that perennial eighteenth-century phenomenon, the participation of the lay public in medical debate. And it raises another problem the medical press had to resolve: that of identity and anonymity.

Ever since Gutenberg, the ethics of attaching names to publications had been ferociously debated. Some deplored the practice as betraying vanity; in genteel circles, it was thought vulgar. Yet, when a man's name was his bond, information without the voucher of a name might command no authority – in particular, it could be thought dishonourable to enter the lists of controversy anonymously, since it precluded a challenge, a point critics made against Lettsom when he sniped at Myersbach from the safety of a shield of pseudonymity.[56]

In the *angina* case, the testimony of the anonymous patient was automatically verified by Heberden (indeed, all papers in *Medical Transactions* were signed, being the work of members of the College). Difficulties of etiquette were sometimes, however, more thorny.

The august College had authority enough to disclaim responsibility for its publication. This was not so easy for a mere editor or a commercial publisher, whose aim was necessarily somewhat different – to create credit *ex nihilo*. Hence anonymous submissions proved a special headache, precisely because the editor was in no position to authenticate the value, the integrity, of the contribution. The editors of the *Medical and Physical Journal* complained that they received articles on 'controversial subjects' signed only with initials, and hence impossible to print. On contentious issues at least, writers must attach their names,[57] insisted the editors, who meanwhile congratulated themselves on the 'great variety of valuable and original communications, authenticated by the respectable signatures of the writers'.[58]

And what of the patients? Did conventional codes protect their identity too? Here practice varied. Patients are commonly identified by some generic description – maybe as a sailor who applied to the hospital; by initials; or by being labelled Mr W——— or Mrs R———. It is not uncommon, however, to find a full name being printed, even in such cases of delicacy as venereal infections. Thus we are told by William Fordyce that a patient of his, 'Mrs Marshall, a carpenter's wife of Long Acre', has painful chancres, and that the case of another, Mr Gordon of Chandos Street, is a 'venereal one'.[59] Class talked: the privilege of privacy was accorded to rank. Within the compass of one single article we not infrequently encounter the full names of lower-class sufferers, while their social superiors are shielded with decorous anonymity. Dr Gourlay discussed the case of 'a young gentleman of family . . . whose name I do not mention for motives of delicacy'.[60] In an assessment of angostura bark, three patients are mentioned, a 'Mr M.', a 'Captain ———' and 'Simon Elliott, a black man'.[61]

Medical periodicals did not evolve inexorably, teleologically, towards the Victorian medical press – which, itself, in any case, was highly variegated. Yet we can see some stages in the development of contents and form. The volumes put out at an early date by societies of gentlemen are, not surprisingly, primarily strings of separate papers, held together by only a contents list and, perhaps, a perfunctory preface. Commercial publications were often similar. Samuel Foart Simmons's *Medical Facts and Observations*, which succeeded his *London Medical Journal* in 1794, contains nothing but cases – some of them original contributions, others reprinted from sources such as the *Philosophical Transactions* and the *Transactions of the Royal Society of Edinburgh*. Simmons claimed such reprinting served the needs of 'persons who are busily employed in the practice of physic', since 'the channels of medical information are now so numerous, and in so many different languages, that many important observations probably remain for a long time unknown'. In any case, the *Transactions* of learned societies were difficult to obtain and beyond people's pockets.[62]

In time, however, a more active, vocal journalistic persona makes itself felt. A good example is offered by the Edinburgh-based *Medical Commentaries*, edited by Andrew Duncan until 1795 when he announced its discontinuation and replacement by the *Annals of Medicine*. An annual, the *Medical Commentaries* claimed to be targeted at a larger public (I presume not specifically professional), and espoused the 'public interest', beneath an epigraph from Baglivi ('*neglecta reducit, sparsa colligit, utilia selegit, necessaria ostendit, sic utile*'). Duncan, who cultivated a certain editorial presence, divided his journal into four sections:

1. 'Accounts of New Books' – impressively meaty abridgements of British and foreign publications, often running, all told, to two hundred pages per issue.

2. 'Medical Observations' – case reports, upon whose 'original' character Duncan insisted.[63]

3. 'Medical News' – a comprehensive listing, sometimes of around eighty pages, including the affairs of medical societies, titles of prize essays, competition winners, news of forthcoming books, obituaries, hospital foundations, advertisements for medical lectures, summaries of university medical courses, medical promotions in the army and navy, reports on the Royal Humane Society, and bits and pieces apparently sent in by readers, for instance, a letter from a Scottish lady reporting a sulphur medicine for gout.[64] Finally,

4. 'A List of New Books'.

Duncan clearly saw himself not just as printing cases but as providing an interesting miscellany and as dealing in news. He sought breadth of coverage, bringing together between two boards matter from the whole medical world ('*sparsa colligit*'). His problem was editorial control. Could all the information that came to hand be trusted? A general disclaimer would have discredited his enterprise, and so he slipped in the occasional individual apologia. Introducing a contribution in the second volume about a woman who voided a snail, he stated that he feared there might be 'deceptions in this story'.[65] Such problems of authentication proved recurrent, leading Duncan to observe in the preface to the sixth volume that 'among the original observations contained in the present volume, there are some which may . . . in some particulars, be founded upon mistaken observation'. Against this, no cast-iron safeguards were possible: 'No one who undertakes the office of a Collector, can be supposed to vouch for the truth of what is merely communicated to him by others. The credit due to such circumstances must, in every instance, depend upon the veracity and discernment of the observer'.[66]

The *Medical and Physical Journal*, which first appeared in March 1799, offers a further instance of a trend towards true journalism. This was significant for being not an annual but a monthly, and its title page boasted that the journal contained 'the earliest information' on medical subjects. Unlike Duncan's annual journal, which, though newsy, was the work of an editor with time to digest his materials, early numbers of the *Medical and Physical Journal* show signs of hasty assemblage against urgent deadlines, with items succeeding each other higgledy-piggledy, and a multitude of bitty fillers penned by the editors, conveying information, abstracting publications, commenting on events and even on other journals.[67] The journalist's preoccupation with speed and punctuality made itself felt. Please date your contributions, begged the editors, so they could be published in strict order of receipt.[68] Consistently with this, the journal had a substantial 'Medical Intelligence' section, called 'Original and Selected', dealing in up-to-the-minute news. Its clinical reports were commensurably brief, occupying only a page or two, by contrast with the twenty- or thirty-page papers common earlier – though they are also sometimes illustrated, even in colour. Turning the pages of the *Medical and Physical Journal*, we sense a new, lively pulse of readers' participation, a talking-shop, self-sustaining in that many items refer back to previous entries. Your last number contained an *apologia* for Brunonianism, complains John Franks in a letter to the editor: please insert the following to redress the balance.[69] Soon a controversy was buzzing in its pages regarding – of all things! – Thomas Beddoes's interpretation of the significance of John Mayow's contribution to the development of English medicine.[70] A sure sign that the *Medical and Physical Journal* had become a high-visibility news-sheet is that Beddoes used it to correct, in double-quick time, an embarrassing blunder in one of his works, where a recipe had given wrong ingredient specifications.[71]

By 1800, what kind of a medical journal could you buy? We have seen the early emergence of collections of case histories by many hands, occasionally published by societies. The country's leading practitioners were clearly eager to publish material in this format, and, doubtless, minor practitioners also sent in their offerings, to get their names into print – a satire published in the *Edinburgh Medical and Surgical Journal* in 1809 told aspiring young doctors to do just that.[72] But the absence of quacks and gross self-publicists is worth noting – the editors of the *Medical and Physical Journal* state that, while wishing to encourage the 'public' and the 'faculty', they had abstained from sending their prospectus to 'empirics'. In fact, the medical press was rapidly becoming a vehicle for anti-quack professional consciousness-raising.[73]

Case histories always remained the staple of the medical journal, but alongside there developed intelligence, book reviews, correspondence columns and other feedback – all in all, an effective talking-shop for the clinical research of the day. The medium was evidently effective in spreading new ideas. Provincial medical societies subscribed to the new medical press. Writing from St Thomas's Hospital around 1800, young Hampton Weekes was constantly telling his father and brother down in the Weald to read the journals: a bit of one-upmanship, but by then also sound advice. 'Every man conversant with the practice of physic', opened a contribution from James Magennis to the *Medical and Physical Journal*,

> must perceive with pleasure the many benefits which are likely to result for the community in general and to the medical profession in particular through the medium of your excellent Miscellany. To the remote country practitioner, cut off from a knowledge of the more recent improvements and discoveries of the capital, it will prove an acquisition of the highest importance . . . it not only conveys a valuable stock of information to all, but likewise serves to stimulate the indolent and awaken a spirit of research in the more learned part of the profession.[74]

Much that is familiar in the best nineteenth-century medical journals was still absent: no editorials, no commentaries upon public events, no causes and crusades, no real sense that the journal is the fourth estate, medicine's public conscience. No sign of Wakley, no Hart, none of the vituperations of the Victorian press. Nevertheless, as Sir Christopher Booth has emphasized, any reader of the journals of the last quarter of the eighteenth century will come away with the feeling that medicine – despite Beddoes's strictures – was moving forward, and that the medical press was becoming Beddoes's 'national bank of medical wealth'.[75] Even more so, he will see signs of a new professional consciousness. Provincial practice in Georgian England spelt isolation and competitiveness. During the next century, the rooting and shooting of the medical press was a prime medium for the attainment of greater collective professional self-consciousness and identity.

Finally: was it a bane or a blessing? The last word goes to Thomas Beddoes, and he was in two minds. He energetically contributed to the genre.[76] But the pressures of print intimidated him, indeed, made him ill. Like Weissmann today, he thought too much was appearing, too fast. '*Did you see the papers today? Have you read the new play – the new poem – the new pamphlet – the last novel?*' was all one heard these days, Beddoes complained. 'You must needs hang your heavy head, and roll your bloodshot eyes over thousands of pages weekly. Of their contents at the week's end, you will know about as much as of a district, through which you have been whirled night and day in the mail-coach'.[77]

Notes

1. Gerald Weissmann (1990) *The Doctor with Two Heads*, New York: Knopf, 135.

2. Thomas Gisborne (1794; ed. cited, 1797) *An Enquiry into the Duties of Men in the Higher and Middle Classes of Society in Great Britain, Resulting from their Respective Stations, Professions and Employments*, 2 vols, London: B. and J. White, ii, 185. See Roy Porter, 'Thomas Gisborne: Physicians, Christians, and Gentlemen', in Roger French, Johanna Geyer-Kordesch and Andrew Wear (eds) (1991) *A History of Medical Ethics*, Cambridge: Cambridge University Press.

3. Gisborne, *An Enquiry into the Duties of Men*, vol. ii, 184. Contemporary priority disputes are discussed in Roy Porter, 'William Hunter: A Surgeon and a Gentleman', in W.F. Bynum and Roy Porter (eds) (1985) *William Hunter and the Eighteenth Century Medical World*, Cambridge: Cambridge University Press, 7–34.

4. Gisborne, *An Enquiry into the Duties of Men*, vol. ii. 184–5.

5. For the rise of scientific and medical publishing in general, see E. Eisenstein (1979) *The Printing Press as an Agent of Change*, 2 vols, Cambridge: Cambridge University Press; John L. Thornton (1966) *Medical Books, Libraries and Collectors: A Study of Bibliography and the Book Trade in Relation to the Medical Sciences*, 2nd ed., London: André Deutsch; A.J. Meadows (ed.) (1979) *The Scientific Journal*, London: ASLIB; David Knight (1975) *Sources for the History of Science, 1660–1914*, London: The Sources of History; *idem*, (1981) *Ordering the World. A History of Classifying Man*, London: Burnett Books. Specifically on handbills, etc, see P. Crawford, 'Printed Advertisements for Women Medical Practitioners in London, 1670–1710', *Society for the Social History of Medicine Bulletin*, xxxv (1984), 66–70. On Culpeper, see Andrew Wear, 'Culpeper and his Tradition', in Roy Porter (ed.) (1991) *Popularizing Medicine*, London: Routledge.

6. D. Kronick (1976) *A History of Scientific and Technical Periodicals: The Origins and Development of the Scientific and Technical Press, 1665–1790*, 2nd edition, Metuchan, N.J.: Scarecrow Press; Roger Hahn (1971) *The Anatomy of a Scientific Institution: The Paris Academy of Sciences, 1666–1803*, Berkeley: University of California Press.

7. (1667) *Philosophical Transactions*, ii, no. 28, 517.

8. Marie Boas Hall (1975) 'The Royal Society's Role in the Diffusion of Knowledge in the Seventeenth Century', *Notes and Records of*

the Royal Society of London, xxix, 173–92; A. Rupert Hall (1974) 'Medicine in the Early Royal Society', in Allen G. Debus (ed.) *Medicine in Seventeenth Century England*, Berkeley: University of California Press, 421–52; *idem* (1971) 'English Medicine in the Royal Society's Correspondence, 1660–1677', *Medical History*, xv, 111–25; Roy Porter (1989) 'The Early Royal Society and the Spread of Medical Knowledge', in Roger French and Andrew Wear (eds) *The Medical Revolution of the Seventeenth Century*, Cambridge: Cambridge University Press, 272–93; Michael Hunter (1981) *Science and Society in Restoration England*, Cambridge: Cambridge University Press; *idem* (1989) *Establishing the New Science: The Experience of the Early Royal Society*, Woodbridge: Boydell and Brewer. For the major role of James Jurin as a collector and distributor of medical information, in respect of smallpox inoculation, see G. Miller (1957) *The Adoption of Inoculation for Smallpox in England and France*, London: Oxford University Press.

9. For the new world of writers see Pat Rogers (1972) *Grub Street: Studies in a Subculture*, London: Methuen; J. Saunders (1964) *The Profession of English Letters*, Toronto: Toronto University Press; A.S. Collins (1927) *Authorship in the Days of Johnson*, Clifton: Augustus M. Kelly; R.L.W. Collison (1973) *The Story of Street Literature: The Forerunner of the Popular Press*, London: Dent; M. Foss (1972) *The Age of Patronage: The Arts in England 1660–1750*, Ithaca: Cornell University Press. A major medical mud-slinging match is surveyed in David Harley, 'Ethics and Dispute Behaviour in the Career of Henry Bracken of Lancaster, Surgeon, Physician and Manmidwife', in Robert Baker, Dorothy Porter and Roy Porter (eds) (1991) *The Codification of Medical Morality in the Eighteenth and Nineteenth Centuries*, vol. i, Dordrecht: Kluwer. For Hunter's elephant folio, see A. Darlington (1986) 'The Teaching of Anatomy and the Royal Academy of Arts 1768–1782', *Journal of Art and Design Education*, v, 263–71; Ludmilla Jordanova, 'Gender, Generation and Science: William Hunter's Obstetrical Atlas', in W.F. Bynum and Roy Porter (eds) (1985) *William Hunter and the Eighteenth Century Medical World* Cambridge: Cambridge University Press, 385–412.

10. Of course, it was mainly quacks and the shadier doctors who got their names in the press. See Roy Porter (1989) *Health for Sale: Quackery in England 1650–1850*, Manchester: Manchester University Press; generally on the rise of the press, see Jeremy Black (1986) *The English Press in the Eighteenth Century*, London: Croom Helm; G.A. Cranfield (1962) *The Development of the Provincial Newspaper 1700–1760*, Westport, Conn.: Greenwood Press; R. Wiles (1965) *Freshest Advices: Early Provincial Newspapers in England*, Columbus: Ohio State University Press; Roy Porter, 'Newspapers as Resources for Social Historians', in I.P. Gibbs (ed.) (1988) *Newspaper Preservation and Access*, Munich: Saur, 84–96.

11. Roy Porter, 'Laymen, Doctors and Medical Knowledge in the Eighteenth Century: The Evidence of the *Gentleman's Magazine*', in Roy Porter (ed.) (1985) *Patients and Practitioners: Lay Perceptions of Medicine in Pre-Industrial Society* Cambridge: Cambridge University Press, 283–314; *idem* (1985) 'Lay Medical Knowledge in the Eighteenth Century: the Case of the *Gentleman's Magazine*', *Medical History*, xxix, 138–68.

These articles contain an extensive bibliography on Georgian periodicals.

At the close of the seventeenth century, John Dunton's various magazines had specialized in answering readers' queries, many medical in nature. See J. Cormick (1973) 'Medical Advice in Seventeenth Century Journalism', *Journal of the American Medical Association*, ccxxiv, 83–6.

12. Indispensable here are W. LeFanu (1984) *British Periodicals of Medicine: A Chronological List*, Oxford: Oxford Wellcome Unit for the History of Medicine; S. Rogal (1980) 'A Checklist of Medical Journals Published in England during the Seventeenth, Eighteenth and Nineteenth Centuries', *British Studies Monitor*, ix, 3–25. See also C. Booth *et al.* (1982) 'Medical Communication: the Old and the New. The Development of Medical Journals in Britain', *British Medical Journal*, cclxxxv, 105–15; Nesta Dean (1955) 'The History of Medical Periodicals', *Oxford Medical School Gazette*, vii, 114–16; N. Howard-Jones (1973) 'Our Medical Literature – Then and Now', *British Journal of Medical Education*, vii, 70–85; F. Garrison (1934) 'The Medical and Scientific Periodicals of the 17th and 18th Centuries', *Bulletin of the Institute of the History of Medicine*, ii, 285–343, updated by David A. Kronick (1958) 'The Fielding H. Garrison List of Medical and Scientific Periodicals of the 17th and 18th Centuries; Addenda and Corrigenda', *Bulletin of the History of Medicine*, xxxii, 456–74.

13. F.N.L. Poynter (1948) 'The First English Medical Journal', *British Medical Journal*, ii, 307–8; P. Johnston-Saint (1938–39) 'The First English Medical Journal', *Medical Press and Circular*, cci, 117–18; Sir Dawson Williams (1928) '*Medicina Curiosa*: An Early Medical Journal', *Glasgow Medical Journal*, cix, 105–9.

14. Thomas Hunt (ed.) (1972) *The Medical Society of London 1773–1973*, London: Heinemann; D'Arcy Power (1939) *British Medical Societies*, London: The Medical Press and Circular.

15. P.J. Bishop (1974) *A Short History of the Royal Humane Society*, London: The Society; E. Thomson (1963) 'The Role of the Physician in Humane Societies of the Eighteenth Century', *Bulletin of the History of Medicine*, xxxvii, 43–51.

16. 'An Earlier British Medical Journal – a Prospectus Issued in 1798', (1936) *British Medical Journal*, ii, 777.

17. At bottom, if at the risk of sounding a little pretentious, one might say that the relations between knowledge and the public constituted the prime issue of the Enlightenment. See Theodor W. Adorno and Max Horkheimer (1972) *Dialectic of Enlightenment*, New York: Herder and Herder; Robert Darnton (1979) *The Business of Enlightenment. A Publishing History of the Encyclopédie, 1775–1800*, Cambridge, Mass.: Harvard University Press; *idem* (1982) *The Literary Underground of the Old Regime*, Cambridge, Mass.: Harvard University Press; Elizabeth Eisenstein, 'On Revolution and the Printed Word', in Roy Porter and Mikuláš Teich (eds) (1986) *Revolution in History*, Cambridge: Cambridge University Press, 186–205; Peter Gay (1971) *The Party of Humanity: Essays in the French Enlightenment*, New York: Norton; *idem* (1956) *Voltaire's Politics: The Poet as Realist*, New York: Vintage; *idem*

(1966–69) *The Enlightenment: An Interpretation*, 2 vols, New York: Vintage.

18. Historians of science have recently been deeply interested in the question of the construction of sources of truth authority by early modern science. See in particular Simon Schaffer (1983) 'Natural Philosophy and Public Spectacle in the Eighteenth Century', *History of Science*, xxi, 1–43; Ian Inkster, 'Culture, Institutions and Urbanity: The Itinerant Science Lecturer in Sheffield 1790–1850', in S. Pollard and C. Holmes (eds) (1976) *Essays in the Economic and Social History of South Yorkshire*, Barnsley: South Yorkshire County Council, 218–32; M. Berman (1978) *Social Change and Scientific Organization: The Royal Institution, 1799–1844*, London: Heinemann Educational; Simon Schaffer, 'The Consuming Flame: Electrical Showmen and Tory Mystics in the World of Goods', in John Brewer and Roy Porter (eds) (1991) *Consumption and the World of Goods*, London: Routledge; S. Shapin and S. Schaffer (1985) *Leviathan and the Air Pump: Hobbes, Boyle and the Experimental Life*, Princeton: Princeton University Press.

19. For the Baconian vision of the triumph of truth, see Charles Webster (1975) *The Great Instauration: Science, Medicine and Reform, 1626–1660* London: Duckworth. Beale to Oldenburg, 21 December 1662, in A.R. Hall and M.B. Hall (eds) (1966–73) *The Correspondence of Henry Oldenburg*, 11 vols, Madison, Wisc.: University of Wisconsin Press, i, 481.

20. Beddoes's criticisms are made mainly in (1793) *A Letter to Erasmus Darwin . . . on a New Method of Treating Pulmonary Consumption, and Some Other Diseases Hitherto Found Incurable*, Bristol: Bulgin & Rosser; *idem* (1799) *Contributions to Physical and Medical Knowledge, Principally from the West of England*, London: T.N. Longman and O. Rees; *idem* (1808) *A Letter to the Right Honourable Sir Joseph Banks . . . on the Causes and Removal of the Prevailing Discontents, Imperfections, and Abuses, in Medicine*, London: Richard Phillips. For discussion, see Roy Porter, 'Thomas Beddoes and the Advancement of Knowledge', in Roy Porter (1991) *Thomas Beddoes: Doctor of Society*, London: Routledge; *idem*, 'Reforming the Patient in the Age of Reform: Thomas Beddoes and Medical Practice', in Roger French and Andrew Wear (eds) (1991) *Medicine in the Age of Reform*, London: Routledge; *idem*, 'Plutus or Hygeia? Thomas Beddoes and Medical Ethics', in Robert Baker, Dorothy Porter and Roy Porter (eds) (1991) *The Codification of Medical Morality in the Eighteenth and Nineteenth Centuries*, vol. i, Dordrecht: Kluwer; *idem*, 'Civilization and Disease: Medical Ideology in the Enlightenment', in J. Black and J. Gregory (eds) (1991) *Culture, Politics and Society in Britain 1660–1800*, Manchester: Manchester University Press, 154–83.

21. T. Beddoes (1793) *A Letter to Erasmus Darwin . . . on a New Method of Treating Pulmonary Consumption, and Some Other Diseases Hitherto Found Incurable*, Bristol: Bulgin & Rosser, 4; see also T. Beddoes (1808) *A Letter to the Right Honourable Sir Joseph Banks . . . on the Causes and Removal of the Prevailing Discontents, Imperfections, and Abuses, in Medicine*, London: Richard Phillips, 92.

22. Beddoes, *A Letter to Banks*, 85.

23. Beddoes (1799) *Contributions to Physical and Medical Knowledge, Principally from the West of England*, London: T.N. Longman and O. Rees, 6.

24. Beddoes, *A Letter to the Right Honourable Sir Joseph Banks*, 82.

25. Beddoes, *A Letter to the Right Honourable Sir Joseph Banks*, 83.

26. Beddoes, *Contributions*, 9.

27. Beddoes, *A Letter to the Right Honourable Sir Joseph Banks*, 93.

28. Beddoes, *A Letter to the Right Honourable Sir Joseph Banks*, 83.

29. Beddoes, *A Letter to the Right Honourable Sir Joseph Banks*, 85.

30. Beddoes (1799) *Contributions to Physical and Medical Knowledge, Principally from the West of England*, London: T.N. Longman and O. Rees.

31. Beddoes, *Contributions*, 9.

32. Questions of confidentiality were debated in such publications as Thomas Percival (1803) *Medical Ethics; or, A Code of Institutes and Precepts Adapted to the Professional Conduct of Physicians and Surgeons*, Manchester: J. Johnson & R. Bickerstaff. See Robert Baker, 'Deciphering Percival's Code', in Robert Baker, Dorothy Porter and Roy Porter (eds) (1991) *The Codification of Medical Morality in the Eighteenth and Nineteenth Centuries*, vol. i, Dordrecht: Kluwer. For the complex assumptions of personal patronage and market individualism shaping medicine at this time, see Dorothy Porter and Roy Porter (1989) *Patient's Progress: Doctors and Doctoring in Eighteenth-Century England*, Cambridge: Polity Press; N. Jewson (1974) 'Medical Knowledge and the Patronage System in Eighteenth Century England', *Sociology*, viii, 369–85; *idem* (1976) 'The Disappearance of the Sick Man from Medical Cosmology, 1770–1870', *Sociology*, x, 225–44.

33. Patients, or their families, particularly wanted to be veiled in privacy in certain medical situations: for example, lunacy, see Roy Porter (1987; paperback edition, Penguin 1990) *Mind Forg'd Manacles: Madness and Psychiatry in England from Restoration to Regency*, London: Athlone Press; and the clandestine delivery of illegitimate babies, see Roy Porter, 'A Touch of Danger: The Man-Midwife as Sexual Predator', in G.S. Rousseau and R. Porter (eds) (1988) *Sexual Underworlds of the Enlightenment*, Manchester: Manchester University Press, 206–32.

34. For this general field see W.F. Bynum and Roy Porter (eds) (1986) *Medical Fringe & Medical Orthodoxy 1750–1850*, London: Croom Helm; Roy Porter (1989) *Health for Sale: Quackery in England 1650–1850*, Manchester: Manchester University Press; R. Cooter (ed.) (1988) *Studies in the History of Alternative Medicine*, London: Macmillan.

35. Roy Porter, 'The Language of Quackery in England, 1660–1800', in P. Burke and R. Porter (eds) (1987) *The Social History of Language*, Cambridge: Cambridge University Press, 73–103.

36. Roy Porter, '"I Think Ye Both Quacks": The Controversy Between Dr Theodor Myersbach and Dr John Coakley Lettsom', in W.F. Bynum and R.S. Porter (eds) (1987) *Medical Fringe and Medical Orthodoxy 1750–1850*, London: Croom Helm, 56–78; J.J. Abraham (1933) *Lettsom: His Life, Times, Friends and Descendants*, London: Heinemann.

37. The concept of public knowledge has been debated in, e.g.,

John Ziman (1968) *Public Knowledge. An Essay Concerning the Social Dimension of Science*, Cambridge: Cambridge University Press.

38. (1765) *Gentleman's Magazine*, xxxv, 524.

39. W. Buchan (1769) *Domestic Medicine, or a Treatise on the Prevention and Cure of Diseases by Regimen and Simple Medicines*, Edinburgh: Balfour, Auld & Smellie; Roy Porter, 'Popular Medicine in Georgian England', in Tim Harris (ed.) (forthcoming) *Popular Culture*, London: Macmillan; *idem*, 'Spreading Medical Enlightenment: The Popularization of Medicine in Georgian England, and its Paradoxes', in Roy Porter (ed.), *The Popularization of Medicine, 1650–1850* (London: Routledge, 1992) which examines Buchan in detail; C. Lawrence (1975) 'William Buchan: Medicine Laid Open', *Medical History*, xix, 20–35; C. Rosenberg (1983) 'Medical Text and Medical Context; Explaining William Buchan's *Domestic Medicine*', *Bulletin of the History of Medicine*, lvii, 22–4.

40. Roy Porter, 'Reforming the Patient: Thomas Beddoes and Medical Reform', in Roger French and Andrew Wear (eds) (1991) *Medicine in the Age of Reform*, London: Routledge. For advice literature see Ginnie Smith, 'Prescribing the Rules of Health: Self-Help and Advice in Late Eighteenth-Century England', in Roy Porter (ed.) (1985) *Patients and Practitioners: Lay Perceptions of Medicine in Pre-industrial Society*, New York: Cambridge University Press, 249–82; *idem* (1985) 'Cleanliness: the Development of an Idea and Practice in Britain 1770–1850', University of London, Ph.D. thesis.

41. David Spadafora (1990) *The Idea of Progress in Eighteenth Century Britain*, New Haven: Yale University Press.

42. Thomas Beddoes (1808) *A Letter to the Right Honourable Sir Joseph Banks . . . on the Causes and Removal of Discontents, Imperfections, and Abuses, in Medicine*, London: Richard Phillips, 130.

43. For discussion of the Georgian medical popularizers see Roy Porter, 'Popular Medicine in Georgian England', in Tim Harris (ed.) (forthcoming) *Popular Culture*, London: Macmillan; *idem*, 'Spreading Medical Enlightenment: The Popularization of Medicine in Georgian England, and its Paradoxes', in Roy Porter (ed.), *The Popularization of Medicine, 1650–1850* (London: Routledge, 1992); C. Lawrence (1975) 'William Buchan: Medicine Laid Open', *Medical History*, xix, 20–35; C. Rosenberg (1983) 'Medical Text and Medical Context; Explaining William Buchan's *Domestic Medicine*', *Bulletin of the History of Medicine*, lvii, 22–4; W. Buchan (1769) *Domestic Medicine, or a Treatise on the Prevention and Cure of Diseases by Regimen and Simple Medicines*, Edinburgh: Balfour, Auld & Smellie. For the perennial accusations against quacks that they were nothing but self-publicizers, see Roy Porter, 'The Language of Quackery in England, 1660–1800', in P. Burke and R. Porter (eds) (1987) *The Social History of Language*, Cambridge: Cambridge Univer- sity Press, 73–103.

44. Roy Porter, 'William Hunter: A Surgeon and a Gentleman', in W.F. Bynum and Roy Porter (eds) (1985) *William Hunter and the Eighteenth Century Medical World*, Cambridge: Cambridge University Press, 7–34. On lectures as property, see S. Lawrence (1985) 'Science

and Medicine at the London Hospitals: The Development of Teaching and Research 1750–1815' Ph.D. thesis, University of Toronto; *idem* (1988) 'Entrepreneurs and Private Enterprise: The Development of Medical Lecturing in London, 1775–1820', *Bulletin of the History of Medicine,* lvii, 171–92; *idem,* 'Educating the Senses: Students, Teachers and Medical Rhetoric in Eighteenth-Century London', in W.F. Bynum and R. Porter (eds) (forthcoming), *Medicine and the Five Senses,* Cambridge: Cambridge University Press; C.J. Lawrence (1984) 'Medicine as Culture: Edinburgh and the Scottish Enlightenment' Ph.D. thesis, University of London.

45. See Roy Porter (1989) *Health for Sale: Quackery in England 1650–1850,* Manchester: Manchester University Press, chs 4 and 7.

46. For these issues, see the discussion in Roy Porter, 'William Hunter: A Surgeon and a Gentleman', in W.F. Bynum and Roy Porter (eds) (1985) *William Hunter and the Eighteenth Century Medical World,* Cambridge: Cambridge University Press, 7–34. It is worth noting that, while head of the Berlin Academy, Maupertuis threatened members with loss of their pensions unless they published. See M. Terrell (1990) 'The Culture of Science in Frederick the Great's Berlin', *History of Science,* xxviii, 333–64.

47. M.J. Peterson (1978) *The Medical Profession in Mid-Victorian London,* Berkeley: University of California Press; Ivan Waddington (1984) *The Medical Profession in the Industrial Revolution,* Dublin: Gill & Macmillan; A.J. Youngson (1979) *The Scientific Revolution in Victorian Medicine,* London: Croom Helm; N. Jewson (1974) 'Medical Knowledge and the Patronage System in Eighteenth Century England', *Sociology,* viii, 369–85.

48. The historical relations of demand and supply in the early consumer society have been the subject of much historical debate. See the 'Introduction' to John Brewer and Roy Porter (eds) (1992) *Consumption and the World of Goods,* London: Routledge.

49. (1757) *Medical Observations and Inquiries,* i, 12.

50. (1769) *Medical Observations and Inquiries,* iii, 7.

51. For instance, William Hunter (1757) 'The History of an Aneurysm of the Aorta, with some Remarks on Aneurysm in General', *Medical Observations and Inquiries,* i, 323–57; and John Fothergill (1757) 'On the Use of the Cortex Peruvianus in Scrophulous Disorders', *Medical Observations and Inquiries,* i, 303–22.

52. (1785) *Medical Transactions Published by the Royal College of Physicians in London,* i. 6.

53. (1785) *Medical Transactions Published by the Royal College of Physicians in London,* i, 9.

54. (1785) 'A Letter to Dr Heberden, Concerning the Angina Pectoris', *Medical Transactions Published by the Royal College of Physicians in London,* iii, 1–11.

55. On the history of the *Critical Review,* see Claude E. Jones (1956) 'The *Critical Review*'s First Thirty Years (1756–1785)', *Notes and Queries,* cci, 678–80; Robert D. Spector (1960) 'The *Monthly* and its Rival', *Bulletin of the New York Public Library,* lxiv, 159–61; Derek Roper (1961)

'The Politics of the *Critical Review*', *Durham University Journal*, liii, 117–22.

56. Roy Porter, '"I Think Ye Both Quacks": The Controversy Between Dr Theodor Myersbach and Dr John Coakley Lettsom', in W.F. Bynum and R.S. Porter (eds) (1987) *Medical Fringe and Medical Orthodoxy 1750–1850*, London: Croom Helm, 56–78. On the wider question of anonymity, see Martha Woodmansee (1984) 'The Genius and the Copyright: Economic and Legal Conditions of the Emergence of the "Author"', *Eighteenth Century Studies*, xvii, 417–32; Walter J. Ong (1979) *Interfaces of the Word: Studies in the Evolution of Consciousness and Culture*, Ithaca: Cornell University Press; *idem* (1982) *Orality and Literacy: The Technologizing of the Word*, London: Methuen; *idem* (1967) *The Presence of the Word: Some Prolegomena for Cultural and Religious History*, New Haven: Yale University Press.

57. (April, 1799) *Medical and Physical Journal*, i, 311. Thomas Bradley 1751–1813 was MD, Edinburgh, 1791 and physician to the Westminster Hospital, 1794–1811, but, according to the *Dictionary of National Biography*, not very successful in his profession.

58. (April, 1799) *Medical and Physical Journal*, i, 312.

59. William Fordyce (1757) 'An Attempt to Discover the Virtues of the Sarsaparilla Root in the Venereal Disease', *Medical Observations and Inquiries*, i, 150.

60. Dr W. Gourlay (for 1791, pub. 1792) 'An Account of the Mineral Waters in the Portuguese Island of St Miguel', *Medical Commentaries*, vi, 232–50, pp. 248–9.

61. Thomas Winterbottom (1794) 'Some Observations Relative to the Angostura Bark', *Medical Facts and Observations*, vi, 41–73, p. 59.

62. (1791) *Medical Facts and Observations*, i, 7.

63. (1786) *Medical Commentaries*, 2nd decade, i, 7. This was published by C. Elliot in Edinburgh, and edited by Andrew Duncan, the Elder (and succeeded by his son of the same name). Duncan was MD St Andrews, 1769, and President of the Edinburgh College of Physicians in 1790, when he obtained the chair of the Institutes of Medicine.

64. *Medical Commentaries*, 2nd decade, i (1786), 392.

65. *Medical Commentaries*, 2nd decade, ii (1788), 395.

66. *Medical Commentaries*, 2nd decade, vi (1792), 6.

67. The boast about 'earliest information' appeared from vol. iii onwards. A controversy is reported from the non-medical (December, 1798) *Monthly Magazine*, on the use of emetics on the apparently dead: (1799) *Medical and Physical Journal*, i, 72.

68. *Medical and Physical Journal*, i (April, 1799), 518.

69. *Medical and Physical Journal*, i (April, 1799), 131.

70. *Medical and Physical Journal*, i (April, 1799), 144.

71. *Medical and Physical Journal*, i (April, 1799), 243.

72. 'Hints to Young Practitioners', *Edinburgh Medical and Surgical Journal*, v (1809), 335–9: 'write monthly reports of diseases in a newspaper or magazine'; quoted in Mary E. Fissell (1991) *The Physic of Charity: Health and Welfare in the West Country, 1690–1810*, Cambridge:

Cambridge University Press, ch. vi, 'Surgeons and the Medicalization of the Hospital'.

73. *Medical and Physical Journal*, i (April, 1799), 311. For anti-quack insertions see i (1799), 337; iii (1801), 435.

74. Arthur Rook (1960) 'General Practice, 1793–1803: The Transactions of a Huntingdonshire Medical Society', *Medical History*, iv, 236–52 and 330–47; J.M.T. Ford (ed.) (1987) *A Medical Student at St Thomas's Hospital, 1801–1802: The Weekes Family Letters, Medical History*, Supplement No. 7, London: Wellcome Institute for the History of Medicine; in a letter of 7 Dec. 1801 (p. 91) Hampton recommends that his brother should search out 'one two or three of the last numbers of the Medical Journal' (probably the *Medical and Physical Journal*) where he can find a case of a woman with a stone; in a letter of 8 Nov. 1802 (p. 231) Hampton tells his father, 'I have taken in ye Medl Journal for this month on account of a Dr Michaelis of Hannover having treated [puerperal fever] successfully by large doses of Opium and Valerian'. For the correspondent (1800) see the *Medical and Physical Journal*, iii, 128–9.

75. Sir Christopher Booth (1987) *Doctors in Science and Society*, London: The Memoir Club, 202–14, 'The Development of Medical Journals in Britain'.

76. It is worth noting that Beddoes used the press to advertise his Pneumatic Institution and to solicit funds for it. See *Medical Commentaries*, viii (for 1793, published 1794), 406.

77. Thomas Beddoes (1802) *Hygëia: or Essays Moral and Medical, on the Causes Affecting the Personal State of our Middling and Affluent Classes*, 3 vols, Bristol: J. Mills, vol. 3, essay ix, p. 163. '*Hypocrite auteur, mon semblable, mon frère*', one is tempted to respond.

2

Periodical knowledge: medical journals and their editors in nineteenth-century Britain

W.F. Bynum and Janice C. Wilson

'Of the making of books there is no end', opined the writer of *Ecclesiastes*, long before the coming of the printing press. At least the medical journal or periodical had the decency to postdate Gutenberg, but it has been apparent for the past couple of centuries that, like books, the making of journals is endless.

Like so much else in medicine, its concepts and institutions, medical journals acquired during the course of the nineteenth century many of the characteristic features which they still possess. In this essay, we examine some of those features of the journals as a group and then, through several selected individual journals, look at the way editorial work fitted into the changing occupational structures and values of the medical profession itself. Our span is 1800 to 1899; that our categorization of types of medical journals bears such a striking resemblance to that devised by the Loudons must be looked upon as an instance of simultaneous discovery, and our charts and tables should be considered as examples of the traditional value of statistics: to demonstrate what the well-trained mind had already grasped intuitively.[1] Anyone interested in medical periodicals in Britain owes an enormous debt to W.R. LeFanu who, at the behest of Fielding H. Garrison and with the encouragement of Sir Humphry Rolleston, published in 1937 his list of periodicals between 1684 and 1899; and a further debt to Jean Loudon and her colleagues at the Wellcome Unit in Oxford, for reprinting it, and updating it with the addition of seventy-three titles to the 738 or so which LeFanu listed. We have found a couple more. LeFanu's bibliography included titles published in Canada, Australia, India and other parts of the British Empire. We have excluded these from our figures, nor have we counted changes in the titles of journals, or journal mergers, to which LeFanu assigned separate numbers. Excluding these, and periodicals founded before 1800, there are left 479 medical periodicals established in nineteenth-century Britain, an average of one about every seventy-seven days.[2] (see Figure 2.1).

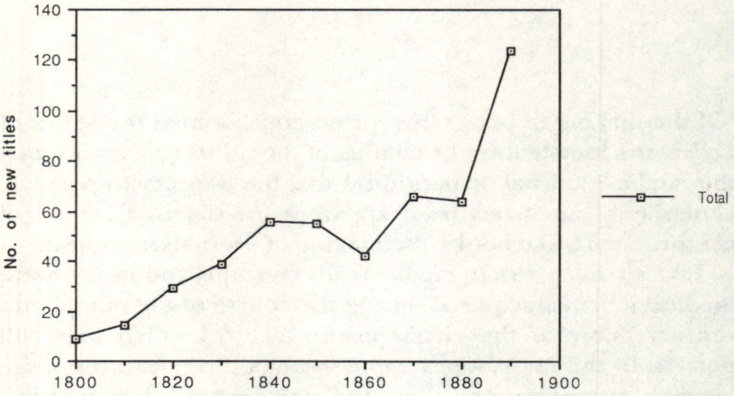

Figure 2.1 Total number of British medical periodicals introduced, 1800–99, by decade. Figures refer forward, i.e. 1800 is for the decade 1800–09

They were not, of course, started at the same rate, but the decadal totals do reveal, in addition to the expected acceleration, a couple of points worth making. In the first place, although a straight line from 1800 to 1890 catches several decades in between, the line is not so steep as Derek Price's work on world scientific periodicals might lead us to expect. Price estimated a hundred-fold increase, from 100 to 10,000, between 1800 and 1900.[3] Figure 2.1 shows newly founded titles, not periodicals actually being published, but the comparable figures of extant periodicals, derived from LeFanu, show that there were 8 in 1800 and 137 in 1900, a seventeen-fold increase. This is not surprising since the scientific community grew during the century at a much faster rate than the medical one.

Slightly more puzzling, perhaps, is the fact that the acceleration was not constant, and new titles actually dropped in the 1860s. We have no ready explanation for this, or indeed for the relative stability of the figures from the 1840s right through to the 1880s. This was, of course, a period of considerable professional consolidation, with the 1858 Medical Act, the development of much more systematic provincial medical education, and the establishment of numerous voluntary and public hospitals and medical societies.[4] On the other hand, as we shall see, the life expectancy of journals increased during the century, the phenomenon picking up pace in the 1840s. Consequently, the number of periodicals actually being produced continued to rise.

In counting, all periodicals are equal, but in reality, of course, they were not. They varied in everything, from cost, format and frequency of publication to targeted audience and philosophical or ideological underpinnings. Our own typology reinforces that of the Loudons, with the addition of a fifth category, the medical science periodical, necessary because of the extension of our analysis up to 1900 (see Figure 2.2).

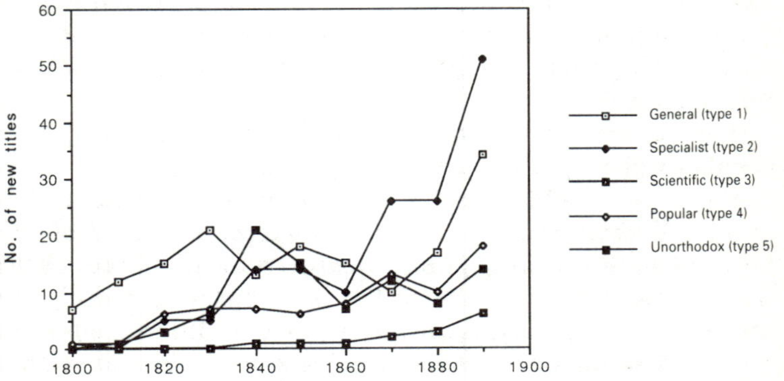

Figure 2.2 Number of new periodical titles introduced in each decade, 1800–99, broken down by type

Roughly, the periodicals can be divided into five classes: first, general periodicals which were aimed at the whole of the medical profession; second, what we have called specialist periodicals the principal readership of which would have been some group within the profession. Thus, a journal which self-consciously sought to reach general practitioners would count as a specialist publication, as would journals aimed at pharmacists, dentists, oculists or psychiatrists. Our third class, the scientific journal, would contain a high proportion of non-clinical material, such as microscopy, anatomy, physiology or bacteriology, although in most cases the readership would have included the scientifically inclined clinician. Between them, these three categories, about two-thirds of the whole, constituted what we can somewhat anachronistically call the professional journal.

Class four, the smallest single group, were those periodicals which disseminated information on health and related topics to the general public, but from the standpoint of orthodox medicine. Several temperance journals fell into this category, as did the short-lived *Anti-tobacco Journal* and some but not all of the journals devoted to diet. About two-thirds of the final category – the unorthodox journals – were concerned with phrenology, homoeopathy or hydropathy. Our attempt to subdivide this group into journals aimed at providers and at consumers of medical care, was unrealistic, despite the fact that a periodical such as the *British Journal of Homoeopathy* was obviously meant for practising homoeopaths. Most, however, seemed more concerned with the believer in the particular system of health and disease being promulgated and make the lay–professional distinction invidious.[5]

The boundaries are not, of course, engraved in stone. The Combes's *Phrenological Journal* could arguably be placed in Class 1, 4 or 5, even if phrenological journals in the latter part of the century became more recognizably heterodox. Some of the periodicals espousing public health reform in the 1840s obviously wanted an informed but partially lay readership; by the end of the century, the leading public health journals were produced primarily for medical officers of health and related professionals, and contain, *inter alia*, a good deal of bacteriology. Journal titles, too, are only a rough guide to their contents. An 1830s periodical called *The Doctor* was a popular magazine; in the 1870s, one with the identical title was for medical practitioners. The *Medical Dispatch* was a professional journal, the

Medical Enquirer a popular one. Two incarnations of a periodical simply called *Health* were orthodox, yet *The Healthian* was unorthodox. A third periodical, entitled *Health*, was one of about ten periodicals with ambiguous titles which we have not been able to examine and was therefore not classified.

Despite these problems, the categories are in most instances sufficiently definite to give the shape of the graph significance. Of note, though not necessarily of surprise, is the fact that specialist journals move from a position of virtual invisibility at the beginning of the century, to lead the field from 1870 onwards. This does not mean that specialty formation was unproblematic in Britain; it continued, in fact, to be resisted by many professional élites long after the turn of the century. Both the impetus and the difficulties are symbolized by the appearance of a journal in 1880 called *The Specialist*. It was devoted to many of the specializations then beginning to emerge: ophthalmology, otology, rhino-laryngology, odontology, dermatology, psychiatry (called psychology in the subtitle) and gynaecology.[6] This was the impetus: the difficulties are encapsulated by the fact that the journal folded after sixteen monthly issues. Other points worth mentioning are that the heyday of the challenge to medical orthodoxy occurred during the 1840s, when that category led the pack before retreating to a poor fourth by the century's end;[7] that general medical periodicals completely dominated the field for the first third of the century; and that scientific periodicals continued to be a poor relation to each of the other types throughout the century, although a similar graph for the present century would undoubtedly show something rather different.

As already mentioned, journal mortality rates remained high throughout the century, although, ironically, more striking improvements occurred earlier in the century than they did for the British population (see Figure 2.3).

The 1810s was the best early decade: 50 per cent of the periodicals founded then lasted for five years or more, a pattern consistently approached if not quite achieved during the middle third of the century. The expansion during the 1820s and 1830s was not notably productive of long-lived journals, despite *The Lancet* of 1823 and the *Glasgow Medical Journal* of 1828. The last two decades were significantly different: by then, well over half of new journals could expect to survive for at least five years, and more than a quarter lasted for fifty years or more.

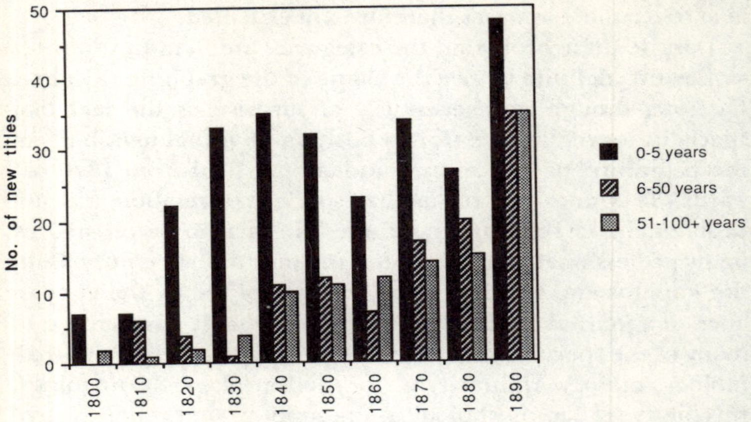

Figure 2.3 Lifespans of all titles introduced, 1800–99, by decade (types 1–5)

In most instances these are still extant. Throughout the century, professional periodicals unsurprisingly stood a better chance of surviving than lay-orientated ones, whether orthodox or not (see Figure 2.4). The former category lasted slightly better than the latter. Only five unorthodox periodicals established during the whole of the century were still being published fifty years after their birth (see Figure 2.5).

Finally, where were these journals published? The statistical answer is both simple and definite: London (see Figure 2.6).

Crudely speaking, during the century, London had 10 per cent of the population and 15 per cent of the doctors. Up to 50 per cent of the profession spent part of their training in the metropolis, almost 75 per cent of the medical journals were published there: about 364 out of 497. Even Edinburgh disappeared as an important centre after the 1820s. The area between the total and the London portion becomes reasonably large during the 1890s, with the birth of several self-consciously local or regional periodicals such as the *Sheffield Medical Journal* or the *Transactions of the North of England Obstetrical and Gynaeco-*

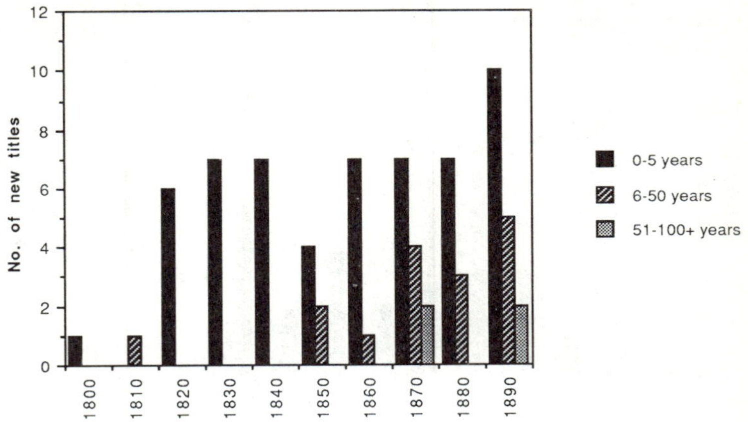

Figure 2.4 Lifespans of orthodox popular medical periodicals (type 4), by decade

logical Society. London was overwhelmingly the centre of medical journal publishing. We have done no further breakdown relating to type of periodical with place of publication, but spot checking suggests that the intuitive feeling that popular and unorthodox journals should be more prominently represented in the provinces, is not borne out. Even Class 4 or Class 5 periodicals were likely to be published in the metropolis.

These, then, are a few general characteristics about a diverse group of periodical publications ranging from shoddy penny weeklies which did not survive more than an issue or two, to lavish, well-illustrated proceedings of élite medical societies. Without editors, no journals, and we shall now look at some aspects of the nineteenth-century medical editor. Dr Johnson saved his wit for the lexicographer, his definition of an editor being merely 'he that revises or prepares any work for publication'. Dr Johnson would not have been surprised to learn that several nineteenth-century medical lexicographers, James Copland (1791-1870), Robley Dunglison (1798-1869), for example, doubled as editors of medical journals as well.[8] Many

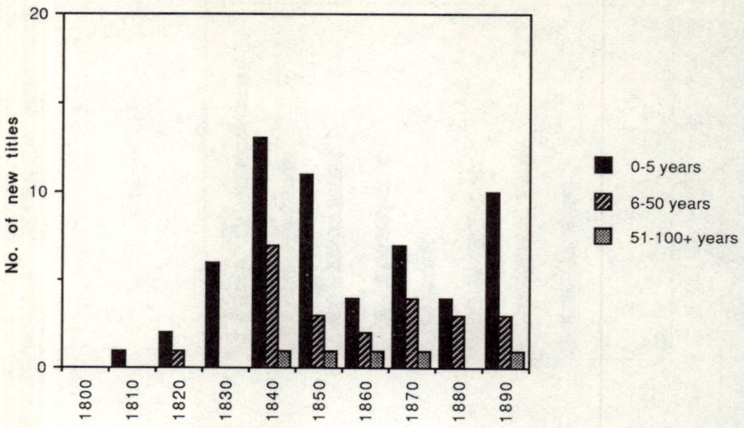

Figure 2.5 Lifespans of unorthodox medical periodicals (type 5), 1800–99, by decade

contributors to periodicals might hold that editors are only half-lexicographers: drudges they may be, harmless they are not.

'Harmless' is certainly not an adjective one would ever associate with the most significant of nineteenth-century medical editors, Thomas Wakley (1795-1862). We cannot recount the well-known story of *The Lancet*, founded by him in 1823, but three brief points are relevant to our analysis of the editorial career. First, Wakley was the first nationally visible medical editor: too visible for many people's tastes. He stamped his journal with his own personality, was exceptionally successful at selling his product and, for the first time, used medical journalism as a platform for the other aspects of his career, including the coronership for Middlesex and a seat in Parliament.

As such, Wakley provided a touchstone, even in some ways, a role model for the competitors who so disliked him and his libellous journal. He did not invent the weekly British medical journal, nor, curiously, was his the first to be born in 1823, since the *Weekly Medico-Chirurgical and Philosophical Magazine* appeared on 8 February, six months before Wakley burst upon

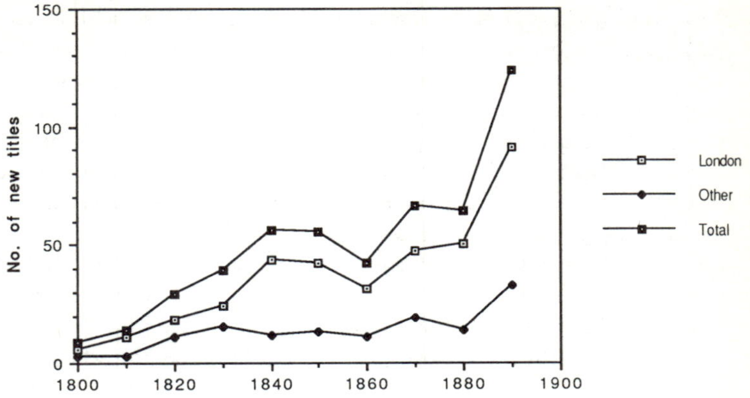

Figure 2.6 London as a place of publication compared to other places in Great Britain, by decade, 1800–99. When two or more locations were listed, the first one only was tabulated

the scene. While this journal did not survive the year, the founding of the *London Medical Gazette* in 1827 was merely the first of several alternatives to *The Lancet.* As Wakley's biographer, Squire Sprigge, put it, rival quarterlies had trouble, since Wakley 'got thirteen shots to one'.[9] More than a dozen weeklies were born in the two decades after 1823, and when the *British and Foreign Medico-Chirurgical Review* took its leave in 1877, after ninety-six years, its lament was:

> For several years we have witnessed the gradual decline in sale of that which once was a good property, and, in spite of all our efforts to infuse new life into our old friend, we have been obliged to stand by and see it languish, so that the period has at last arrived when to continue to publish it would be to incur an annual loss which would rather increase than diminish as time went on. The reason of all this is that the day for quarterlies is gone by, and, in the face of the daily and weekly periodicals, a quarterly, with

> its thoughtful articles and well-digested reviews, is no longer appreciated as formerly.[10]

The weekly format suited Wakley's aims perfectly, which, as a final point, were to *reform* as well as simply inform. Frequent publication gave time and space for leaders, correspondence and political comment. It created the potential for the medical journal to be an instrument of reform in ways that quarterlies or even monthlies could never have aspired to. This is not to say that there had been no crusading medical editors before Wakley, nor that improvement and professional consolidation had been absent from earlier journal agendas. But Wakley carried the reforming journal on to a new plane, thereby demonstrating how potent a force the periodical could be.

Wakley was *sui generis*: even Ernest Hart (1835–98), that other great reforming editor of the century, was not quite in the same mould.[11] Besides, as we shall see, editing, then as now, was the primary occupation for only a fraction of those involved in producing medical journals. As a principal career, medical journalism has never been the joy – or burden – for more than a few, and this was certainly so in nineteenth-century Britain. Nevertheless, there are some patterns to the medical editorial career in Victorian Britain, and it is to these that we now turn.

Edward Gibbon would have described the attempt to discover all of the several thousand individuals involved in the editorial process for all nineteenth-century medical journals as of antiquarian but not necessarily historical merit. We have confined ourselves to a non-random sample of some twenty professional journals, i.e. drawn from our Classes 1, 2 or 3. Popular and unorthodox periodicals would also repay analysis but would, we believe, raise rather different issues. However, one lay-orientated journal – *The Doctor* – was included, since the title did not make its tone or content very clear. A list and brief histories of all the journals examined are included in the Appendix.

For the most part, we selected journals with good survival rates, although the *Edinburgh Medical Journal* and the *Medical Press and Circular* (Class 1 periodicals) both serve as salutary reminders that no journal, even after 200 years, can be assured of immortality. Both have recently gone under. Our small sample also demonstrates the bibliographical jungle which journals can be. The *Edinburgh Medical Journal* was created in

1855, by the amalgamation of the *Edinburgh Medical and Surgical Journal* and the *Monthly Journal of Medicine.* Ancestors of the former went back, under four titles, to 1733; the latter had had two other names since its birth in 1841 and had in addition absorbed in 1846 the *Northern Journal of Medicine.*

Nine journal titles make up the prehistory of the *British and Foreign Medico-Chirurgical Review,* which acquired that name in 1848. The *Dublin Medical Press* lasted for almost a century after combining with the *Medical Circular* in 1865; it moved its office to London and lost the 'Dublin' in the title. More often than not, name changes signalled changes in editors, and amalgamations are almost a guarantee of declining circulation, financial or other difficulty.[12]

Our specialist journals include two short-lived ones and three which have presumably had telegrams from the Queen. Significantly, perhaps, the two casualties, the *Annals of Military and Naval Surgery and Tropical Medicine* and the boldly-entitled *The Specialist,* were one-man bands, the former anonymously edited by someone back in London on sick leave, the latter by a Sheffield aurist, Herbert Junius Hardwicke, who had studied in Germany. Its early demise suggests that it was rather ahead of its time and that, in any case, the heterogeneous collection of clinical specialisms it embraced had little in common beyond the fact that they were beginning to merge as specialisms. The other specialist journals illustrate the other side of the coin. The *Asylum Journal of Mental Science* (now the *British Journal of Psychiatry)* was associated from the beginning with a parent society; *Brain,* founded by a distinguished quartet of psychiatrists and neurologists, was adopted in its tenth year as the organ of the Neurological Society of London; the *British Journal of Dermatology* had an independent existence until 1922, when it became the official organ of the British Association of Dermatology and Syphilology.[13]

In a contemporary classification, *Brain* would almost certainly count as a scientific publication. Our three scientific journals point towards stages in the development of what was the most successful British medical science in the century, physiology. The *London Physiological Journal* was in fact devoted to microscopy and edited by S.J. Goodfellow and Edwin Quekett, assisted, as the title page had it, by 'many eminent observers'. It survived for a mere five issues and Quekett himself died young three years later.[14] Histology was a kind of half-way house between anatomy and physiology, taught in the middle decades of the century by those who were increasingly concerning themselves with issues of function. Nevertheless, it was unexceptional for anatomy and physiology still to be combined, as they were, in a journal of that title, established in 1866 by the surgeon–anatomist (Sir) George Humphry and the anatomist (Sir) William Turner, and edited by them and three others.[15] Two physiology editors were added in 1875, with the deliberate intention of giving more space to physiology. By then, however, one of the physiology editors, Michael Foster, was dissatisfied for physiology to remain as anatomy's poor relation, and the *Journal of Physiology*, started by him in 1878, placed an emphasis on experimental work from the beginning.[16] The *Journal of Anatomy and Physiology* eventually lost 'physiology' from its title, though not before it became associated with the Anatomical Society of Great Britain and Ireland, established in 1887; an arrangement made easier by the fact that Humphry was the Society's first president.[17] The *Journal of Physiology* was acquired by the Physiological Society only in 1926, after J.N. Langley's death, though from its fourth volume it had published the Society's proceedings.[18]

This brief account of most of the twenty periodicals on which we have concentrated should already have indicated some of the different characteristics of the various kinds of journals. For each of them we have assembled biographical details of the editors, throughout the nineteenth-century life of the journal. This has involved about 175 individuals, with connections ranging from sole editor and proprietor, to the much remoter function of membership on an editorial board, the duties of which were never publicly stated. The result is nothing so systematic as a prosopography, but it does permit us to make a few generalizations about the nineteenth-century medical editor.

The first point is the obvious one: medical journalism and medical editing were not defined careers. We chose several weeklies in the hope that some forgotten Wakleys or Harts might turn up: men who earned their living (or at least most of it) from their editorial work. From our sample, this is simply not the case: Arthur Jacob and Henry Mansell edited the *Dublin Medical Press* for twenty-one years, but combined it with ophthalmological and obstetrical work respectively.[19] George Ross was a London general practitioner as well as co-founder and sole editor for thirteen years of the *Medical Press and Circular*.[20] The first full-time editor of the monthly journal *The Practitioner* was William Thomson, appointed in the 1950s, when the journal was in its ninth decade.[21] The financial reasons are obvious: most periodicals would not generate enough income to support the luxury of a full-time editor.

The economic may not be the entire answer, however, for occupational pluralism was a central feature of medical life in Victorian Britain and, for the vast majority of men, success in clinical practice was the yardstick by which their fellows measured them.[22] For most of the century, the vast majority of hospital consultants, clinical and basic science teachers, medical officers of health, poor-law medical officers, port-authority and prison doctors, also kept their hand in private practice. It took courage not to, and courage, too, to fight for full-time salaried positions within the state, local authority or public health sectors. With so many of the élites to be counted among those with lucrative private consultancy work, the assumption was easily made that those who could, became consultants, and those who couldn't, became panel doctors, medical officers of health or asylum superintendents. Or medical editors. Thus, it could be argued that editors brought the prestige of their hospital appointments and addresses of their private consulting rooms to their duties. This is true in some instances, but our sample suggests something rather more subtle.

First, it suggests that, as a group, editors, co-editors, assistant editors and editorial board members constituted on the whole an ambitious crew. To be sure, the journals we have examined are not among the most obscure; but it is striking how many men who ultimately achieved professional success in medicine had editorial stints in their backgrounds. Among our sample might be mentioned the physicians Sir Robert Christison, Sir John Forbes, Alfred Swaine Taylor, John Hughes Bennett, Sir Thomas Lauder Brunton and Sir Edward Sieveking; among the surgeons, Sir Thomas Spencer Wells and Sir Jonathan Hutchinson. Most of these appear in our cohort by virtue of editorial experience relatively early in their careers, before honours, presidencies and knighthoods. Even Hutchinson, contained in our counting only by virtue of membership on the large editorial board of the *British Journal of Dermatology*, had much earlier spent a year as editor of the *British Medical Journal*, and was a long-time moving force behind another periodical series which appears in LeFanu, the monographs of the New

Sydenham Society.[23] Like Sir Benjamin Ward Richardson, another Victorian eccentric, Hutchinson also edited his own journal, to which he was the sole contributor.[24]

In short, the career profiles of many of our men suggest that medical journalism was a means, not an end: a stepping stone, not the culmination of their aspirations. Typically, a four-to-ten-year stint as an editor in early-mid career is the pattern. Editors lasting for more than ten years are the exception rather than the rule; as are editors taking on time-consuming duties after their late 30s or early 40s. Take, for instance, John Conolly, or William Benjamin Carpenter, or E.A. Parkes: each put in three-to-five-year periods editing the *British and Foreign Medico-Chirurgical Review*, while angling for something better, such as (in Conolly's case) the superintendency at Hanwell Asylum.[25] In other instances, editing provided not so much a stepping stone as a safety net: a way to earn money while attempting to rebuild a career. Conolly, in fact, turned to editing and writing after his disastrous time as Professor of Medicine at University College; Robert Knox served his time with the *Medical Times* while fleeing from the traumas of the Burke and Hare scandal in Edinburgh, and there are suggestions that Marshall Hall spent a brief and completely unsuccessful period with the *Medical Times*, at the height of his disputes with the Royal Society about his neuro-physiological experiments.[26]

That we have no more than a hint of Hall's association with the periodical reminds us that the cloak of anonymity that we associate with the great Victorian quarterlies extended to the more highbrow medical periodicals. Leaders, reviews and commentary were routinely unsigned, and even the name of the editor or editorial board is sometimes difficult to find. This is in marked contrast with George Shipman's journal, *The Doctor*, which he edited between 1833 and 1837. Aimed at families, his periodical extolled the virtue of his own remedies and reminded readers that 'the Editor of *The Doctor* may be personally consulted every Monday, Wednesday and Friday evening from 5 till 8 o'clock, at 4, Broadway, Ludgate Hill, near Apothecaries Hall. Fee 2s 6d'. Shipman was no quack, simply a general practitioner with fairly down-market aspirations.[27]

The rewards of working with journals which took themselves seriously – and wished their readers to do likewise – were more subtle than free advertising for the editor. The economics of medical publishing is a topic which has proved fairly elusive, but where established publishers were involved, such as Churchill, Macmillan or Longman, editorial payments were certainly common if not universal, and it is difficult not to conclude that the financial incentives were extremely important for editors still not firmly established in their practices. Ideas for new journals presumably originated sometimes with the publisher, sometimes with the would-be editor. Sharp publishers could be on the look-out for new journals. When, in 1837, William Sherwood, the publisher of the *British and Foreign Medical Review*, died, John Churchill proposed himself to its editor, John Forbes, as a suitable alternative. By the next year, Churchill was its publisher, paying Forbes £25 an issue to edit it. The change in publisher obviously worked, since Forbes gave up a lucrative practice in Chichester in 1840, to move to a London practice and easier association with the journal.[28]

Wakley apart, the more élite general medical periodicals of the earlier period can be seen as in many ways attempting to mirror the forms, formalities and conventions of the great Victorian quarterlies.[29] As the more specialist and scientific periodicals became more important in the second half of the century, this began to change. We can describe this transformation in terms of two trends: a switch from editorial individualism to editorial collectivism in the production of journals; and a growing emphasis on professional rather than economic gains on offer to the editor.

Both of these trends are most strikingly associated with the linking of journals with professional bodies or institutions. This was no new phenomenon: the *Medical Essays and Observations* of 1733 were published by 'a Society in Edinburgh'. Furthermore, throughout the century, most new journals were independently established, the private property of either the publisher or the editor. Foster and then Langley owned the *Journal of Physiology*, even after it was loosely affiliated with the Physiological Society. Even so, a large number of the Class 1 periodicals born in the last third of the century were based within a hospital, a medical school or medical society; Class 2 journals were frequently the result of collective activity of specialist societies such as the Association of Medical Officers of Health, or the Society for the Study and Care of Inebriety; Class 3 periodicals often originated in departments, such as the physiology departments at Cambridge or Owens College, Manchester, or the Thompson Yates Laboratories in Liverpool. With this came the more common appearance of editorial boards, the possibility of some form of informal peer review, and the probability of a more open editorial policy and more shared responsibility.[30]

There were losses, perhaps, as well as gains. It may be more fun to read the racier style of the early numbers of *The Lancet* or even the altogether more sober *Medical Times*, than an issue of the *Journal of Pathology and Bacteriology*. And we can certainly exaggerate the extent to which the safeguards that are supposed to guarantee fairness and accuracy in modern scientific and medical journals were in place by the end of the century. Nevertheless, editorial boards gave the appearance of objectivity and respectability, even if they were sometimes no more than so much window dressing. At the very least, it is easier by the century's end to find out who the editors actually were, even if the daily routine which actually produced the finished product remains a mystery.

Appendix

Brief publishing histories of 17 nineteenth-century British medical professional periodicals, for which prosopographical data on editors were analysed. Periodicals are listed chronologically within each category. An open entry indicates the periodical is extant. (Source: W.R. LeFanu, *British Periodicals of Medicine: A Chronological List 1640–1899*, revised edition, Oxford: Wellcome Unit for the History of Medicine, 1984)

Category 1: General professional periodicals

Medical Essays and Observations, 1733–44; continued as Essays and Observations, 1754–65; continued as Medical and Philosophical Commentaries, 1773–95; continued as Annals of Medicine, 1796–1804; continued as Edinburgh Medical and Surgical Journal, 1805–55; merged with Monthly Journal of Medicine (continuation of [The London and Edinburgh] Monthly Journal of Medical Science, 1841–55, which incorporated Northern Journal of Medicine, 1844–46) to form Edinburgh Medical Journal, 1855–1955.

London Medical Journal, 1781–90; continued as Medical Facts and Observations, 1791–1800; continued as Medical and

Physical Journal, 1799–1814; continued as London Medical and Physical Journal, 1815–33; continued as Medical Quarterly Review, 1833–35; continued as British and Foreign Medical Review, 1836–47; joined with Medico-Chirurgical Review, 1824–47 (continuation of Medico-Chirurgical Review and Journal of Medical Sciences, 1820–24; which was a continuation of Medico-Chirurgical Journal, 1818–20) to form British and Foreign Medico-Chirurgical Review, 1848–77.

London Medical, Surgical and Pharmaceutical Repository, 1814; continued as London Medical Repository, Monthly Journal and Review, 1814–28; continued as London Medical and Surgical Journal, 1828–37.

London Medical Gazette, 1827–51, joined with Medical Times, 1839–51 to form Medical Times and Gazette, 1852–85.

Dublin Medical Press, 1839–65, joined with Medical Circular, 1852–65 to form Medical Press and Circular, 1866–1961.

Retrospect of Practical Medicine and Surgery, 1840–45; continued as Retrospect of Medicine, 1846–1901.

The Doctor (Category 4: Orthodox Popular Journals), 1832–37.

The Doctor, 1871–78.

Practitioner, 1868– .

Category 2: Specialist professional periodicals

Asylum Journal of Mental Science, 1853–58; continued as Journal of Mental Science, 1858–1962; continued as British Journal of Psychiatry, 1963– .

Annals of Military and Naval Surgery and Tropical Medicine and Hygiene, 1863.

Brain, 1878– .

Specialist, 1880–81.

British Journal of Dermatology, 1888– .

Category 3: Scientific professional periodicals

London Physiological Journal, 1843–44.

Journal of Anatomy and Physiology, 1866–1916; continued as Journal of Anatomy, 1916/17– .

Journal of Physiology, 1878– .

Notes

1. Of particular background relevance to the themes of this essay is John L. Thornton, *Medical Books, Libraries and Collectors*, 2nd, revised edn., London: André Deutsch, 1966, esp. chapters 8 ('The Growth of Medical Periodical Literature') and 11 ('Medical Publishing and Bookselling').

2. W.F. LeFanu, *British Periodicals of Medicine. A Chronological List, 1640–1899*, revised edn. (ed. J. Loudon), Oxford: Wellcome Unit for the History of Medicine, 1984; Samuel Rogal, 'A Checklist of Journals Published in England During the Seventeenth, Eighteenth and Nineteenth Centuries', *British Studies Monitor*, 1980, *9* (3) 3–25.

3. Derek J. de Solla Price, *Little Science, Big Science*, New York: Columbia University Press, 1965, 8–9.

4. On professional developments during the century, cf. Irvine Loudon, *Medical Care and the General Practitioner*, Oxford: OUP, 1986; Jeanne Peterson, *The Medical Profession in Mid-Victorian London*, Berkeley: University of California Press, 1978; Geoffrey Rivett, *The Development of the London Hospital System 1823–1982*, London: King Edward's Hospital Fund for London, 1986.

5. Roy Porter, *Health for Sale: Quackery in England, 1660–1850*, Manchester and New York: Manchester University Press, 1989; W.F. Bynum and Roy Porter (eds), *Medical Fringe and Medical Orthodoxy*, London: Croom Helm, 1987; Roger Cooter (ed.), *Studies in the History of Alternative Medicine*, Basingstoke: Macmillan in association with St Anthony's College, Oxford, 1988.

6. For Victorian comment on specialism, cf. J. Russell Reynolds, 'Specialism in Medicine', in *idem*, *Essays and Addresses*, London: Macmillan, 1896. For modern comment, see Peterson, *Medical Profession* (note 4), 247–59, 272–9.

7. cf. Logie Barrow, 'Why Were Most Medical Heretics at Their Most Confident Around the 1840s? (The Other Side of Mid-Victorian Medicine)' in Roger French and Andrew Wear (eds), *British Medicine in an Age of Reform*, London: Routledge, 1991.

8. Biographical details of both are in *Dictionary of National Biography* (*DNB*). Dunglison was briefly associated with the *London Medical Repository* before emigrating to the United States, where he had a very successful career as a medical teacher and author. There are also accounts of his life in *Dictionary of American Biography* and *Dictionary of Scientific Biography*.

9. S. Squire Sprigge, *The Life and Times of Thomas Wakley*, London: Longmans, Green and Co., 1898, p. 163; cf. Mary Bostetter, 'The Journalism of Thomas Wakley' in J.H. Wiener (ed.) *Innovators and Preachers: The Role of the Editor in Victorian England*, Westport, Conn: Greenwood Press, 1985, 275–92.

10. 'Publisher's Notice' in Volume LX (1877) of the *British and Foreign Medico-Chirurgical Review*.

11. See Peter Bartrip's essay in this volume and his *Mirror of Medicine, A History of the BMJ*, Oxford: Clarendon Press, 1990.

12. 'Introductory', the Editors [G.A. Gibson, Alexis Thomson and Harvey Littlejohn], *Edinburgh Medical Journal*, N.S. *17* (1905), 1–9, for a brief history of that journal and its editors until the late nineteenth century; for a history of the *Medical Press and Circular*, see Robert J. Rowlette, *Medical Press and Circular 1839–1939: A Hundred Years in the Life of a Medical Journal*, London: Medical Press and Circular, 1939; and 'Death of a Weekly Journal', *BMJ* 1961 (ii), 949.

13. For *Brain*, cf. W.F. Bynum, 'The Nervous Patient in Eighteenth- and Nineteenth-Century Britain: The Psychiatric Origins of British Neurology', in W.F. Bynum, Roy Porter and Michael Shepherd (eds), *The Anatomy of Madness*, vol. i, London: Tavistock, 1985, 89–102; and R.A. Henson, 'The Editors of *Brain*', *The Practitioner 221* (1978), 639–44.

14. Goodfellow (1809–95) subsequently became a consultant physician to the Middlesex Hospital and an expert in 'nervous and hysterical disorders' (*Munk's Roll, IV*, 79–80). Quekett's short career is summarized in the *DNB*.

15. William Turner, 'Preface to the Fortieth Volume', *Journal of Anatomy and Physiology 40* (1905–6), v–viii; E.W. Walls, 'The Journal of Anatomy, 1867–1966; Volume 100' *Journal of Anatomy 100* (1966), 1–4. For Turner and Humphry, see *DNB*.

16. Gerald L. Geison, *Michael Foster and the Cambridge School of Physiology*, Princeton: PUP, 1978, 187–8, 300–1.

17. E. Barclay-Smith, *The First Fifty Years of The Anatomical Society of Great Britain and Ireland: A Retrospect*, London: John Roberts Press Ltd, 1937.

18. Edward Sharpey-Schafer, *History of the Physiological Society During its First Fifty Years, 1876–1926*, Cambridge: CUP, 1927; W.F. Bynum, 'A Short History of the Physiological Society, 1926–1976', *Journal of Physiology 263* (1976), 23–72.

19. For Jacob (1790–1874), see *DNB*. For Mansell (1806–79), see *BMJ* 1879 (ii), 554; and Rowlette, *Medical Press* (note 12), 2–8.

20. For Ross (1815–75), cf. Rowlette, *Medical Press* (note 12), 67ff, and *BMJ* (1975) ii, 445–6.

21. The first editor of *The Practitioner*, Francis Anstie (1833–74), had been on *The Lancet* staff before becoming an editor himself. Sir Humphry Rolleston, 'History of *The Practitioner*', *Practitioner 150* (1944), 321–8; 'Centenary of *The Practitioner*', *New England Journal of Medicine 279* (1968), 42–3.

22. One of us (WFB) has examined some aspects of this phenomenon in an essay entitled 'Medical Values in a Commercial Age', in T.C. Smout (ed.), *Victorian Values: Proceedings of Joint British Academy and Royal Society of Edinburgh Conference*, Oxford, Published for the British Academy by OUP, forthcoming.

23. G.G Meynell, *The Two Sydenham Societies: A History and Bibliography of the Medical Classics Published by the Sydenham Society and the New Sydenham Society (1844–1911)*, Acrise, Kent: Winterdown Books, 1985.

24. Herbert Hutchinson, *Jonathan Hutchinson, Life and Letters*, London: William Heinemann, 1946; Arthur Salusbury MacNalty, *A*

Biography of Sir Benjamin Ward Richardson, London: Harvey & Blythe, 1950.

25. The most recent analysis of Conolly's rather chequered career fails to mention his three-year stint with the periodical (1836–39), which coincided with the nadir of his fortunes: Andrew Scull, 'A Victorian Alienist: John Conolly, FRCP, DCL (1794–1866)', in W.F. Bynum, *et al.*, *The Anatomy of Madness* (note 13), I, 103–50.

26. The evidence for Hall is circumstantial: the preface to Volume 6 (1842) of the *Medical Times* mentions that the editor or editors have served 'our first year's stewardship'. The preface to Volume 7 (1843) refers to 'the wanton and unprincipled personalities of the persons who preceded us in the case of this Journal . . .', and goes on to say that 'Dr Hall treated us in it [the transaction of the journal] with an ill usage only second to that with which he has been accustomed to treat himself'. It is possible, but unlikely, that another Dr Hall was involved. No biographer has mentioned the episode, but his wife Charlotte, who published a full-length life in 1861, eschewed material which would have cast him in a bad light.

27. Victor G. Plarr, 'An Early Victorian Medical Journal', *BMJ*, 1925 (i), 1101; S. Wood, 'The Doctor, 1832–37', *Medicine Illustrated VII* (1953), 500–1; and the essay by Michael Harris in this volume.

28. Correspondence between Churchill and Forbes in Longman Archives, vol. 57, Copy Letterbooks, 1834–1856, pp. 56 and 115, British Library.

29. Walter E. Houghton (ed.), *The Wellesley Index to Victorian Periodicals, 1824–1900*, Toronto: University of Toronto Press, 1966; Richard D. Altick, *The English Common Reader: A Social History of the Mass Reading Public 1800–1900*, Chicago: University of Chicago Press, 1957.

30. For peer review, see Stephen Lock, *A Difficult Balance: Editorial Peer Review in Medicine*, London: Nuffield Provincial Hospitals Trust, 1985; John C. Burnham, 'The Evolution of Editorial Peer Review', *Journal of the American Medical Association*, vol. 263, Jan–June 1990, 1323–29.

3

Medicine, politics and the medical periodical 1800–50

Jean Loudon and Irvine Loudon

Today, when the excessive number of medical journals is a common source of complaint it is salutary to realize that even by the end of the eighteenth century some were voicing the same concern.[1] This was why the editors of the *Medical and Physical Journal* excused the introduction of yet another periodical by saying in 1800 that the state of science 'gives us a good claim to our expectations' of improving communication and the healing art.[2]

There was indeed an explosive growth. Figure 3.1 charts some of the features of the medical periodicals which were established between 1800 and 1849. Each periodical is represented by a numbered line or a cross. A cross indicates a journal which died in its first year; a line represents length of life. Change of title is indicated by a vertical bar and change of number; an upturned arrow shows that the journal amalgamated with another. The numbers are those used in the chronological list of British medical periodicals by William LeFanu, on which the whole of Figure 3.1 and much of this essay is based.[3]

The total is 168 (not including changes of name), an average of just over three new periodicals a year. The rate at which they were established was more or less steady, with only a few periods such as 1828–39 when the rate increased to just over four a year. One of the most surprising features is how many were ephemeral. Table 3.1 gives the details, and shows that nearly three-quarters failed to survive for twenty or more years and most of them died in infancy. Only twelve (7.1 per cent) survived to the twentieth century. Between 1825 and 1839, no less 47.5 per cent died in their first year, and 21.5 per cent (making 69 per cent in all) failed to reach their second birthday.

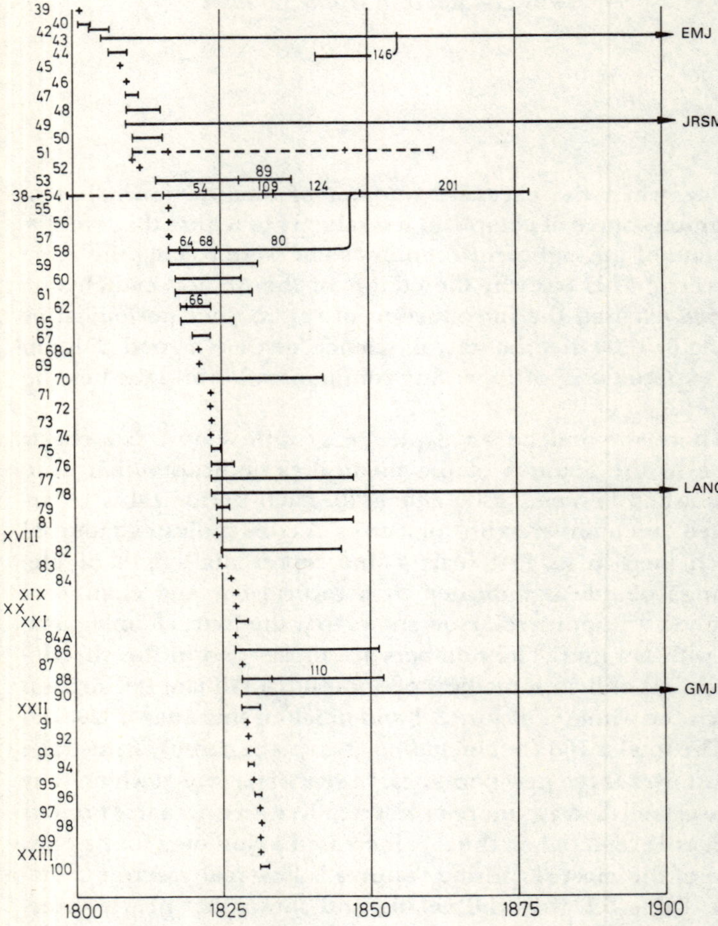

Figure 3.1 **Features of medical periodicals established 1800–49**

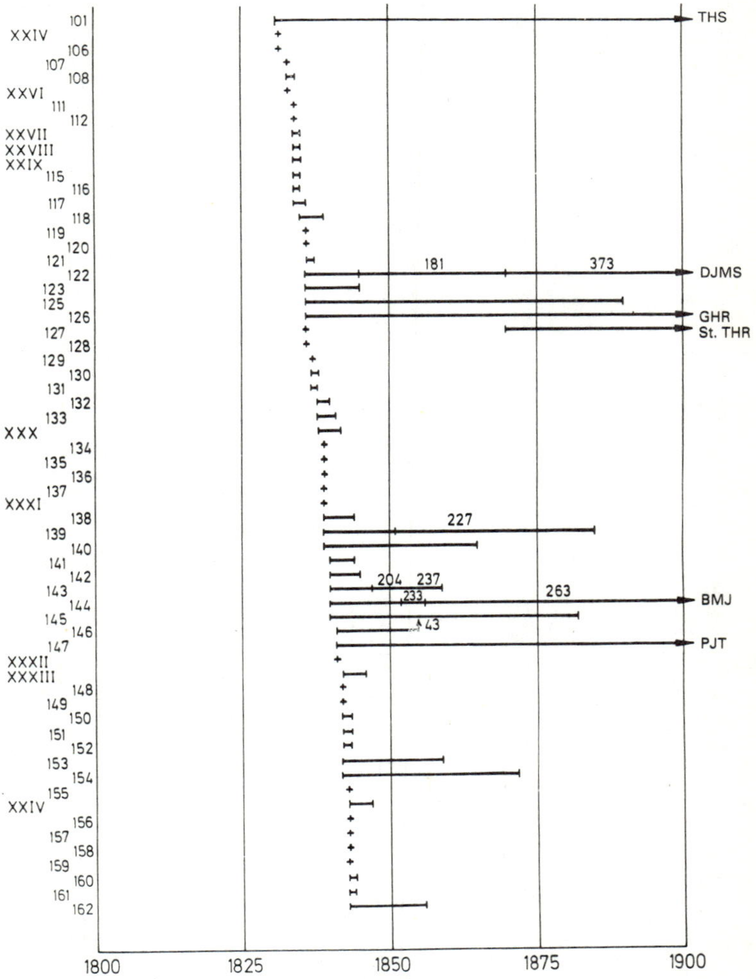

Figure 3.1 continued

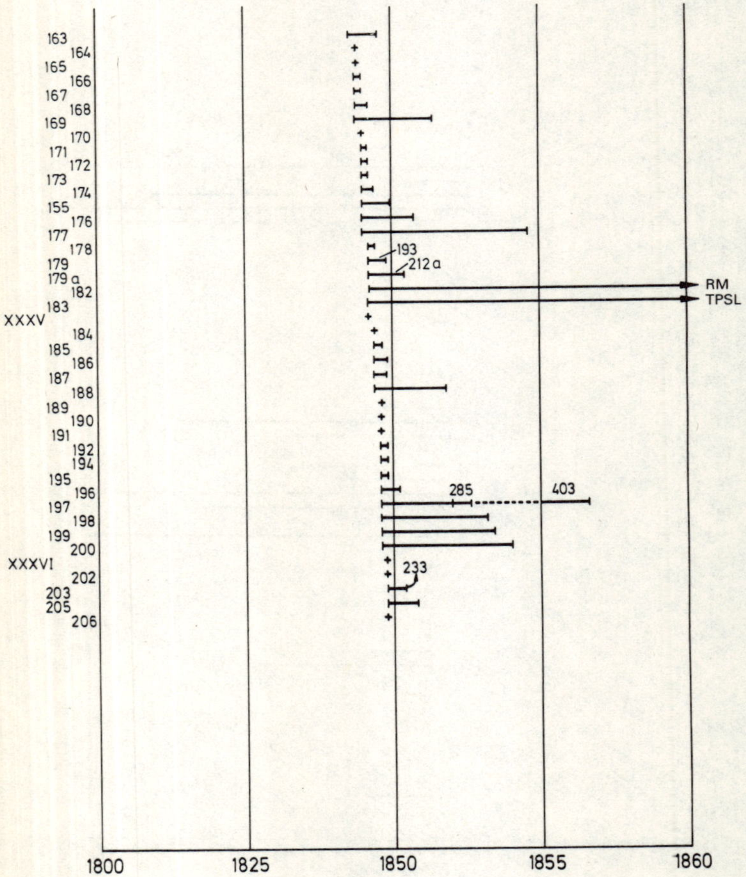

Figure 3.1 continued

For explanation see text. The journals which were still being published in the twentieth century were as follows: EMJ, *Edinburgh Medical Journal.* JRSM, *Journal of the Royal Society of Medicine. Lancet.* GMJ, *Glasgow Medical Journal.* THS, *Transactions of the Hunterian Society.* DJMS, *Dublin Journal of Medical Science.* GHR, *Guy's Hospital Reports.* St. THR, *St Thomas's Hospital Reports.* BMJ, *British Medical Journal.* PJT, *Pharmaceutical Journal and Transactions.* RM, *Retrospect of Medicine.* TPSL, *Transactions of the Pathological Society of London.*

Table 3.1 Length of survival of the 168 British medical periodicals established between the years 1800 and 1849 (inclusive)

Period of survival	*Number*	*Percentage of total*
1 year or less	63	37.5
Over 1 year but less than 5 years	44	26.2
Over 5 years but less than 20 years	16	9.5
Total number surviving for less than twenty years	123	73.2
Survived into the twentieth century	12	7.1

Source: Figure 3.1

As one might guess, not all were orthodox medical journals. In fact, the phrase used by Cassedy, 'health-related journals', is probably a better description of these periodicals than 'medical journals'.[4] Table 3.2 has information on this point. Unlike Table 3.1 and Figure 3.1, Table 3.2 includes periodicals established in the eighteenth and surviving into the nineteenth century. There were 181, divided as follows, although it should be said that the classification was not easy and edges of the divisions were often blurred. 'Mainstream medicine' indicates journals which dealt with most or all branches of orthodox medicine. 'Orthodox specialist' consists of journals devoted to single subjects such as chemistry, pharmacy, anatomy, public health, dentistry and pharmacology. The 'fringe' or unorthodox journals were concerned mainly with mesmerism, phrenology and homoeopathy, and the remainder, loosely categorized as 'other', consists of a variety including some journals which were patently self-advertisement, and several which were designed to educate the public on medical matters. The relative proportions can be seen in Table 3.2 which shows that the category with the best chance of survival was the 'specialist orthodox' periodical, while the 'other' category had the worst chance. The survival rate of 'mainstream medicine' was only marginally better than that of 'fringe medicine'.

Table 3.2 The division, according to type, of all medical periodicals established between 1800 and 1850 (inclusive) as well as those established in the eighteenth century which survived into the nineteenth

*Type of periodical**	*Number*	*Percentage of total*	*Percentage surviving for 1 year or less*
Total	181	100.0	36.5
Mainstream medicine	95	52.4	35.7
Orthodox specialist	37	20.4	24.3
'Fringe'	24	13.2	33.3
Other	25	13.8	60.0

*For descriptions of terms see text.

Why did some periodicals die early, while others survived? Obvious answers are dull contents, poor editing, bad business sense and lack of money in a world of gross overproduction. An important factor, too, was ownership and editorship, and on this basis medical periodicals can be divided into three groups. First, those which were privately owned but had various editors, for example the *Medical and Physical Journal*. Second, those in which the owner and editor were the same person, at any rate initially; examples are James Johnson's *Medico-Chirurgical Review*, Thomas Wakley's *Lancet* and George Man Burrows' *London Medical Repository*. Third, the reports or transactions of institutions of one kind or another: medical societies, associations, colleges and hospitals, which for convenience we have labelled 'house journals'.

One of the finest of all the early journals, the *Edinburgh Medical and Surgical Journal*, was really a house journal, for it was supported by the Edinburgh College of Physicians and its editor, Andrew Duncan junior, professor of the Institutes of Medicine in the University of Edinburgh, was almost the only editor to hold a senior appointment. Apart from the *British Medical Journal*, the most famous house journal which still survives today is the *Journal of the Royal Society of Medicine*, established in 1809 as the *Medico-Chirurgical Transactions* and renamed the *Proceedings of the Royal Society of Medicine* in 1907.[5] It was always a prestigious journal, and probably the only one within our period which refereed papers submitted for publication.[6]

House journals possessed the obvious advantage that members of the institution could be counted on to write articles and act as a captive readership willing, and able, to underwrite at least some of the cost of publication. Nevertheless, the output of house journals was sometimes sporadic. The *St. Thomas's Hospital Reports* first appeared in 1836, slept like Rip van Winkle, and woke up to appear regularly after 1870. The episodic nature of the *Transactions of the Royal College of Physicians*, which produced only six volumes between 1768 and 1820, provoked a characteristically tart comment from the *Edinburgh Medical and Surgical Journal*. When Volume 4 of the *Transactions* appeared in 1813, Edinburgh remarked that:

> The College now and then finds a little leisure, and now and then feels a little zeal, for the cultivation of medical science. These paroxysms of exertion occur, it is true, but seldom and at distant periods, like the visits of the influenza, and their exciting causes are not always discernible by the multitude. 250 years had passed away . . . when the first fit came on and the first volume of its *Transactions* was published in 1768 . . . and now after the silent lapse of 28 years more, the 4th volume comes forth . . . [It is] not as good as *Medical Essays* of Edinburgh or *Medical Observations and Inquiries* of London . . . The inferior merit of the present volume will not admit of dispute . . .

That put the London physicians in their place. For good measure, Edinburgh remarked that the new volume of the *Transactions* used 'large portions of paper by means of type of unusual size and small pages'.[7]

Aims, prices, costs and profits

New journals usually began with a statement of aims. Almost without exception they wished to promote the 'healing art', and provide a continuing education for doctors who might have little time or money for books. The healing art covered both case histories and more fundamental enquiries, often, as in the eighteenth century, taking the form of 'letters' or 'communications'. Vaccination, the work of Hodgkin and Bright, anaesthesia, and changing attitudes to mental illness and public health are all recorded in the journals. Editors were, however, increasingly aware of the anecdotal and, by implication, possibly unreliable nature of much published case material; but enough of the better sort was not always available.[8] Generous space was given to lengthy digests and reviews of books and periodicals. A surprisingly large number (up to 50 per cent) of the 'critical analyses' were of books and periodicals published abroad.[9] In addition, most journals gave about a tenth of their space at the end to medical intelligence, news of societies, lectures in London and Edinburgh, obituaries, and general items – meteorology, topography and travel and so forth.

Although refereeing was apparently negligible, 'obnoxious' and scurrilous contributions were regularly declined. Articles we would call 'prurient' decrease in number. Increasingly, anonymity was disallowed and footnoted references given in published articles. Indexes for the mainstream journals were comprehensive. The effect of all this was to promote the sense of corporate professionalism that lay behind the movement for the reform of medical education and practice that took place from 1812 to 1858.

There were less overt aims. The move for an educated profession involved strong attacks on quackery and the exclusive London Royal Colleges. If a journal was successful it made money for owners, and advertisement, even fame and professional advancement, for its editors.[10] Why, when the competition was so intense, did so many men attempt to establish a new medical periodical? A glance at Figure 3.1 suggests that betting on horses or greyhounds would have been a safer investment. Billings (somewhat unfairly) observed in the United States that it was 'as useless to advise a man who was determined to do so not to start a medical journal as it is to advise him not to commit suicide' because:

> The prevailing motivation behind such rash undertakings was not the scientific spirit. Nor was it the urge for direct profit, but as an indirect advertisement, or – and this is more common – the desire to have a place in which the editor can speak his mind and attack his enemies without restraint.[11]

Some publishers had influence on policy. Richard Phillips owned the *Medical and Physical Journal* and was also the founder–owner of the *Monthly Magazine*.[12] A colourful character, a radical and a republican, Phillips personified the cross-connections between the lay and medical periodical press. Phillips encouraged medical reform, was antagonistic towards the Royal Colleges in London, and thus supported the emerging general practitioners. He showed early concern for the medical welfare of the poor and, more unusually, he supported vegetarianism and a humanitarian attitude towards animals.[13]

As Roy Porter has pointed out more than once, medicine was not a closed shop in the 'long eighteenth century', but a subject for open discourse between educated laymen and doctors.[14] Indeed, the first editor of the *Monthly Magazine* was a medical practitioner, John Aikin, who published lists of the diseases seen at the hospitals and dispensaries, lists which were also a regular feature in medical periodicals. Thus it was reasonable to suppose that if there were a market for lay periodicals, there should be a market for medical ones, not least because of the growth of general practice and the consequent hunger for sources of medical information beyond the text books. There is evidence too that laymen, clergy and others, read the medical periodicals.

Perhaps the most powerful force behind the rapid growth of medical journals in the nineteenth century was the huge expansion of the general press whose influence is evident in the best, or at least the most successful, of the early nineteenth-century periodicals. They combined scientific papers of the kind found in house journals with a lay magazine format. The *Edinburgh Medical and Surgical Journal* and the *Medical and Physical Journal* did this, publishing scientific papers and editorials on medical science alongside medical politics, reviews, correspondence, news, obituaries, and notices of lectures and societies. Lists of books and journals received appeared regularly, together with notices to correspondents which seemed to take the place of answering letters. Letters from correspondents appeared only occasionally, and there was no general 'letters to the editor' section as understood today.

Although the broad resemblance to modern medical journals is often quite striking, there was one marked difference. Nineteenth-century medical journals tended to reprint information or whole articles from other publications, and this included journals published in Europe, India and occasionally the US. This was not regarded as plagiarism or breach of copyright. On the contrary, it was a kind of compliment. Articles from *The Lancet* were hardly ever reprinted as a sign of disapproval at *The Lancet*'s bad manners.

The high early mortality of medical periodicals suggests it was not easy to make ends meet. What, then, was their price, and what did they cost to produce? Table 3.3 shows the actual prices of a small selection of medical periodicals and the equivalent prices today.[15]

Clearly, high-quality mainstream periodicals were not cheap. A year's subscription equalled the cost of one standard textbook (£1–£2). Unfortunately we know very little about the costs of production, still less about circulation. According to Johnson, the cost in 1822–23 of producing one number of his quarterly *Medico-Chirurgical Review* was £100 and the cost of paper and printing was 9 shillings a page in the first volume in 1820.[16] Sales had risen from an initial 200 copies in 1820 to 1575 copies in 1822–23, producing a revenue of £340 5s, plus £23 10s from advertisements, for each quarterly number.[17] The profit after expenses was around £260 a quarter. It may well be that Johnson was a sound business man, for with becoming modesty he wrote that the journal brought him an annual income of £1000: the 'whole history of periodical medicine has exhibited not a single instance of individual success, or independence from such a source alone'.[18] This was not in fact true. The *London Medical Repository* was certainly profitable for George Man Burrows.[19]

Unfortunately, the *Edinburgh Medical and Surgical Journal* loftily avoids cost and profits, but it is unlikely the Edinburgh College of Physicians was any the poorer for producing such a widely read journal. The *Medical and Physical Journal* was unspecific about circulation, but suggested that sales of the first two numbers 'exceeded considerably that of any medical journal hitherto published'. There is some evidence of a circulation war in 1814–15, when malicious rumours circulated that the

Table 3.3 The prices of a selection of medical periodicals in the first half of the nineteenth century. A rough estimate of the equivalent price today is given in brackets below each quoted price (for the basis of this estimation see Note 15).

Periodical	*Frequency of publication*	*Cost of each number*	*Cost per year*
Mainstream medical journals			
Medical and Physical Journal			
Initial price in 1800	Monthly	1s (£2.50)	12s (£30)
Price raised in 1802			15s 6d (£38.75)
Price of all 19 vols in 1808			13 guineas (£682.50)
'Bargain offer' of 19 vols: 1808			£10 (£500)
London Medical Repository			
Price in 1816	Monthly	2s 6d (£6.24)	30s (£75)
Edinburgh Medical and Surgical Journal			
Price in 1823	Quarterly	6s (£15)	24s (£60)
Lancet			
Price in first half of 19th C.	Weekly	6d (£1.25)	26s (£65.00)
Medico-Chirurgical Review			
Price in the 1820s	Quarterly	4s6d (£11.25)	18s (£45)
Monthly Medical Record			
1842: lasted only six months	Monthly	8d (£1.66)	
Journal of Public Health			
1847–49	Monthly	1s (£2.50)	
Medical journals for the public			
The Medical Adviser and Guide to Health and Long Life			
(1823–25)	Weekly	1d (20.8p)	
The Doctor. A medical Penny Magazine			
(1832–35)	Weekly	1d (20.8p)	
The People's Medical Journal and Family Physician			
(1850–51)	Weekly	3d (62.4p)	

Medical and Physical Journal had ceased publication. By 1815, however, its orders were said to be 'increasing'.[20] There were, then, enough successful journals to tempt new venturers; but all in all it was very difficult to make a go of a medical periodical as a private financial venture. Much depended on the character and energy of the owner and editor. The outstanding example, of course, is *The Lancet.*

The character and contents of medical periodicals

Compared with the general periodical press, the medical press was on the whole polite and dispassionate. The *Medical and Physical Journal* with its cool analytical approach to medical politics stood head and shoulders above most anti-establishment journals, such as the poorly produced *Monthly Gazette of Health* (1816–31), a little known and rather disreputable journal which published scurrilous attacks on physicians and the Royal Colleges, and saw itself as the supporter of the rank and file.[21]

The *Edinburgh Medical and Surgical Journal* was studious and gentlemanly. It was much more than a local Scottish journal, but often stressed the superiority of Scottish medicine, pointing out that Scotland did not recognize divisions in the profession to anything like the same extent as England. All practitioners in Scotland, including the physicians, were the general medical attendants to their patients. The licentiates of the Edinburgh College of Surgeons:

> are qualified to practise medicine, surgery, and midwifery, in all their departments and even pharmacy; and the result is that we hear no complaints in the whole of Scotland about the merely nominal distinctions of physicians, surgeons, and surgeon–apothecaries.[22]

Slightly snooty in tone, this journal rarely missed an opportunity to swipe at London and remind it that Edinburgh was the Athens of the North and the cradle of the most advanced doctors and medical opinions in the world. It scorned the Association of Apothecaries and Surgeon–Apothecaries, a group to which we come later. It thought less than nothing of the London Royal College of Physicians, but so did a lot of sensible people.[23] It was firmly believed, and not without reason, that Edinburgh always managed things better. It was always said that Edinburgh was 'cliquey', and it showed. As far as its medical journal was concerned, Glasgow, Aberdeen and St Andrews might scarcely have existed.[24]

Taking the medical press before 1823 as a whole, however, although there were criticisms of colleges and institutions, by the standards of the time it was characterized as basically well-informed but tame.[25] Tame, that is, until the publication in 1823 of *The Lancet* by its inimitable and partisan editor, Thomas Wakley, who was to the medical establishment of the 1820s and 1830s what *Private Eye* is to the political and social establishment today. That acute observer of the medical scene, James Fernandez Clarke (who, incidentally, worked for *The Lancet*), believed that Wakley had introduced a sea-change in medical periodicals:

> The Medical press was, previous to the establishment of the *Lancet*, conducted, at all events, with a gentlemanly spirit, and with becoming deference to Professional opinions and views. It was, in many instances, tame, but, as a rule, not ill-informed, and had scrupulously avoided all *personal* matters. It remained for the *Lancet* to introduce into Medical journalism an element which has caused more heart-burning and quarrels than any other could possibly have done. This was the system of personal attack and the calling of nicknames.[26]

Clarke believed that Wakley modelled himself on Cobbett and wanted to be seen as a radical. While Clarke excused Cobbett's virulent attacks on the ground that politicians were fair game:

> There was no excuse for Wakley. He entered into the fight against men from whom he had received no injury, and with whom he had had no previous quarrel . . . he attacked them personally; called Hospital Surgeons "bats", and Scotch Doctors "dubs". He abused them in a spirit of ridicule . . . the *Lancet*, as representative of Medical literature, was sunk so low that it was only to be classed with the very lowest of the political prints of the day. At this time the Medical press had obtained an unenviable notoriety for its personal abuse and the low *morale* which it manifested.[27]

Wakley used the bludgeon, not the rapier. His crude and often puerile attacks on medical men and medical corporations, at first amusing, soon become tedious. All the same, whether you supported or hated Wakley, you could not deny the high standard of production of his journal, nor the excellence of many of its articles on medicine and medical science as well as medical politics. Indeed, it had few equals before 1850 and by that time, if not before, Wakley regretted his early excesses and 'conducted the journal associated with his name with so much good feeling (and, I may say, with proper dignity), as to have made amends for the past'. As Clarke says, 'Mr Wakley's undoubted shrewdness and ability' were never in question.[28]

What were the contents and quality of these journals? Here we can take only a brief glance. The *Medico-Chirurgical Transactions* stood out for the high scientific quality of its papers relating to medical practice, and its excellence was acknowledged by other journals which regularly condensed and copied its papers. Many are still quoted today.[29] Typically there were up to 28 papers of about 24 pages each in a volume of 680 pages.

An analysis of the contents of the first twenty volumes of the *Edinburgh Medical and Surgical Journal* based on counting columns in the cumulative index, showed that fevers easily came first, occupying 16 complete index columns. This was followed by pharmacology (8); other forms of therapy (venesection, hot and cold water and so on) (6); consumption/phthisis, lungs and respiration (4); smallpox and vaccination (3); and three each on a wide variety of other medical and surgical conditions. Neither public health nor mental disease achieved a full column entry. A similar survey of the *Medical and Physical Journal* for the twenty years 1799–1818 showed 86 index columns devoted to diseases, 43 to scientific experiments, 22 to physiology and 21 to reports of societies.

What is, perhaps, unexpected is the internationalism of these journals. They listed a large number of foreign 'periodicals received' and combed them for extracts which they believed would interest their readers, producing articles and critical analyses on clinical and biomedical topics, natural history, travel and topography world-wide, but especially Europe, West Africa, India and North America. The *Edinburgh Medical and Surgical Journal* and the *British and Foreign Medical Review* (later the *British and Foreign Medical and Surgical Review*) were prime examples.[30] The end of hostilities in Europe in 1815 was widely welcomed in the medical press, although material from Europe had most notably been published all the time (as it was from the US in times of war with Britain). Communication became easier and facilitated one of the most striking and unexpected features of medical journalism in the period 1800–1850: its internationalism.

Medical journals, medical politics and medical reform

There was a reciprocal relationship between medical reform and the medical periodicals. They stimulated and nurtured each other throughout the period of medical reform from the late eighteenth century to the Medical Act of 1858.

The origins of medical reform were complex and have been described by one of us elsewhere.[31] But the main features are clear. The aims of reform were to introduce a national system of formal education, examination and registration of all medical practitioners and thereby create a unified profession, not only to improve the state of medicine, but also to enable the public to differentiate between the orthodox and the unorthodox medical practitioners, the regulars and the quacks, the true and the false. Quackery included not only the blacksmiths, butchers and other tradesmen who treated fractures and fevers, but even more the chemists and druggists who set themselves up as doctors, and the multitude of 'ignorant midwives' who delivered babies; all these must be outlawed, partly through legal sanctions, but largely by the public which, when it was provided with certified and properly trained regular practitioners, would desert the quacks in droves and go to the regulars; or so they thought, wrongly as it happens.

The Colleges of Physicians and Surgeons saw no need for reform of themselves. The physicians, who had their system of examination for the licentiate and election to the fellowship of the London College, were complacently satisfied with the practice of physic as it was and always had been and even maintained that their authority extended throughout England. The parvenu College of Surgeons had its examination for membership. Although this was open to all practitioners (and as such was an excellent source of revenue) the College had one aim only: to create an élite of 'pure surgeons' which would place the surgeons on a par with the physicians and well above the rabble of general practitioners. The only group which needed, and indeed desired, extensive reform was the rank and file of the profession, the general practitioners who constituted over 90 per cent of all medical practitioners and, incidentally, the majority of the readership of mainstream medical journals.

Today, when the GP is so flooded with material that stories of medical journals unopened or consigned to the waste-paper basket are commonplace, it may be difficult to appreciate the hunger for medical knowledge in the early 1800s. The surgeon–apothecary/general practitioners at the turn of the century were not, as often portrayed in the past, ignorant illiterate tradesmen of quasi-professional status. There were some like that, but more often they were, by the standards of their time, capable, educated and even cultivated men earning a good professional income. Their training consisted of apprenticeship combined in many instances with voluntary attendance at courses on anatomy, surgery, physic, pharmacy and midwifery at hospitals or private medical schools. For such as these the medical periodicals with their extensive coverage of new books were a vital source of medical knowledge and new ideas. They were the market for which the *London Medical, Surgical and Pharmaceutical Repository: Monthly Journal and Review* was established in 1814 with the specific purpose of bringing new theory and practice to country practitioners.[32] But the medical periodicals served another purpose of great importance: they fostered the new and growing sense of corporate identity amongst general practitioners.

The eighteenth-century surgeon–apothecaries were very parochial. Locally they might be people of substance, but their interests seldom extended far beyond the nearest large town. They knew the practices of neighbouring medical men and occasionally heard with awe of the vast fees charged by doctors in London, but that was another world. They owed nothing to and thought even less of the London medical corporations and had no sense of belonging to a national group within a united profession. All this was to change in the early nineteenth century. Medical reform was in the air from the time that Edward Harrison, MD (Edin.) of Horncastle in Lincolnshire produced his comprehensive plan for the reform of medical practice.[33]

Although there was much good sense in Harrison's plans, they were crushed by the Royal College of Physicians who would not countenance the idea of reform initiated by someone who was not a member of the College and, worse still, an Edinburgh graduate. Medical reform came to the forefront again with the famous meeting of some 200 medical men in July 1812, which took place in the Crown and Anchor tavern in the Strand and was attended by those who were 'the first in rank, ability and character amongst the London practitioners'.[34] At this meeting the Association of Apothecaries and Surgeon–Apothecaries was established. It drew up plans and prepared Bills which led ultimately to the flawed Apothecaries Act of 1815.

The Association of Apothecaries and Surgeon–Apothecaries (later to become the Associated General Practitioners) began as a London affair and rapidly expanded to the provinces. In all this, periodicals played a vital part.[35] They published the proceedings of the Association, listed the membership which encouraged others to join in, and provided the medium through which general practitioners developed a new sense of belonging to a country-wide group with common aims and ideals. They also provided the means whereby medical practitioners who would never have dreamt of writing a book could publish their views on the state of medicine or give accounts of epidemics or medical cases.[36]

It would be wholly mistaken, however, to suppose that medical reform followed a path of smooth upwardly mobile progress towards a better, amicable and unified medical profession. On the contrary, it was characterized by an unparalleled degree of intra-professional strife as the general practitioners sought to raise themselves to a dominant position and the Colleges of Physicians and Surgeons made sure they did not. Much of the strife was mediated through the columns of the medical periodicals which are almost the only source on what really happened in the period of medical reform.[37]

The roles and reactions of the periodicals varied widely. We have touched on this, noting the general aloofness of the *Edinburgh Medical and Surgical Journal*, which behaved like an outsider looking in, jibbing at the daftness and pettiness of English medical arguments. We have noted the comprehensive and balanced approach of the *Medical and Physical Journal*, and also the *London Medical Repository* under the editorship of the President of the Association of Apothecaries and Surgeon–Apothecaries; and the raucousness of organs such as the *Gazette of Health*. *The Lancet* had a lot to say but not to much purpose. Wakley disliked the term 'general practitioner' but he positively loathed the College of Surgeons for its nepotism and élitism. He wanted general practitioners to be called surgeons, and he used the struggles of the general practitioners so blatantly as an opportunity to attack the medical corporations that his contributions to the debate were nullified. The *Transactions of the Associated Apothecaries* provide the only comprehensive account of events preceding and immediately following the Apothecaries Act of 1815, and the *British Medical Journal* and its predecessors are an invaluable source on the conflicts which preceded the Medical Act of 1858. Possibly with *The Lancet* in mind, the *British Medical Journal* trod gingerly on medical reform, anxious not to offend the medical corporations.

It is impossible here to explore all the attitudes of the medical periodicals to medical politics and medical reform; but enough has been said to underline the vital importance of the medical periodicals not only in presenting new ideas on medical practice and medical research, but also in reflecting and shaping the development of medical education and the medical profession. If they fulfil all those roles today, they learnt their trade in the first half of the nineteenth century. That was their formative period.

Notes

1. A. Rook, 'General practice 1793–1803: The Transactions of a Huntingdonshire Medical Society, part II', *Medical History*, 1960, 4: 330–47, 344.

2. *Medical and Physical Journal*, 1800, 4: preface.

3. W.R. LeFanu, *British periodicals of medicine. A chronological list, 1640–1899*, revised edition (ed. J. Loudon), Oxford: Wellcome Unit for the History of Medicine, 1984. Periodicals in the additional appendix are indicated in Figure 3.1 by Roman numerals.

4. There has been remarkably little written in Britain about medical periodicals, and nothing to compare with J.H. Cassedy, 'The flourishing and character of early American medical journalism, 1797–1860', *Journal of the History of Medicine and Allied Sciences*, 1983, 38: 135–50.

5. When it changed its name in 1907, it incorporated a number of other periodicals, notably the *Transactions of the Pathological Society of London* (founded in 1846) which was published thereafter as the Section of Pathology in the *Proceedings of the Royal Society of Medicine*, and the *Transactions of the Obstetrical Society of London*, a marvellously rich and informative periodical established in 1859 which became the Section of Obstetrics and Gynaecology and was never quite the same again.

6. In 1843, twenty-four Fellows of the Society were elected by Council to referee papers submitted for publication. There were many distinguished names including Thomas Addison and Richard Bright of Guy's Hospital, J. Arnott, J. Bostock and G.M. Burrows, the surgeon Robert Ferguson and the well-known London obstetricians Robert Lee and Sam Merriman. *Medico-Chirurgical Transactions*, 1843, 26: iv.

7. *Edinburgh Medical and Surgical Journal*, 1814, 10: 104–16.

8. The *Edinburgh Medical and Surgical Journal*, 1810, 6: 493 in commenting on the first number of the *Medico-Chirurgical Transactions* noted that there were not enough first-rate articles so 'we must be contented with inferior excellencies'.

9. The *Medico-Chirurgical Review* consisted wholly of review articles, resembling a *Reader's Digest* of medicine. It published no original articles. It was a genuine review, expressly aimed at those with little time, money or opportunity, deliberately rejecting the 'mystic reveries of German incubation', the 'pedantic display of names without things, references without quotations, or quotations without use'. (1820, 1: preface and p. 138; 1821–2, 2: 906; and 1824, 5[ns 1]: preface).

10. Andrew Duncan refers regularly to his prospects of promotion in the *Edinburgh Medical and Surgical Journal*. John Conolly was an esteemed editor of the *London Medical Repository* and the *British and Foreign Medical Review*. In the popular medical press, editors frequently give their addresses and consulting hours, for example Thomas Harrison Yeoman in *The People's Medical Journal and Family Physician* 1850–1.

11. Billings's wry comment was written in 1879. The quotations are taken from J. Cassedy, 1983, p. 150. See note 4.

12. See the *Medical and Physical Journal*, 1812, 27: 1 where Phillips said the journal was planned in 1797 and that previously medical periodicals suffered from 'temporary or inadequate support'.

13. On animals this journal expressed disgust at the cruel nature of physiological experiments carried out by the French (1815, 33: 401) and stressed 'the necessity of weighing well the objects in view' before animal experiments were undertaken (1816, 35: 460–1). It suggested experiments on living animals were only justifiable for tests of poisons (1817, 37: 110–12) and it defended the harmless hedgehog that does *not* steal milk from cows (1817, 38: 431).

14. See *The Gentleman's Magazine* and F.H. Garrison, 'Medicine in the *Tatler*, *Spectator* and *Guardian*', *Bulletin of the Institute of the History of Medicine* 1934 2: 477–503, especially pp. 478–9.

15. For today's equivalent prices we have used the crude but simple process of multiplying prices by 50. We do so on the grounds that the available income of the average GP of the 1970s or early 1980s after tax and expenses was usually around £15,000, while that of his predecessor in the period 1800–50 was probably around £300. It is of course impossible in any field accurately to translate nineteenth-century incomes, costs and prices into today's equivalents when financial circumstances are so very different. One of the major difficulties here is the very wide range of general practitioners' incomes in the first half

of the nineteenth century: from a low level of £150–200 a year (£7,500 to £10,000 today) to well over £1,000 a year (£50,000). See I. Loudon, *Medical Care and the General Practitioner*, Oxford: OUP, 1986.

16. *Medico-Chirurgical Review*, 1820, 1: 551.

17. *Medico-Chirurgical Review*, 1822–3, 3: preface.

18. ibid.

19. Obituary notice of G.M. Burrows, *Medical Directory*, 1847, 189–93.

20. See *Medical and Physical Journal*, 1814, 31: 176; 1815, 33: 344; 1815, 34: 1.

21. A later version of the same was the *Medical Record* of 1842 which only lasted six months, was published by an association of medical reformers, and attacked the Home Secretary, Sir James Graham, and the Royal Colleges.

22. *Edinburgh Medical and Surgical Journal*, 1824, 22: 162–3.

23. There is a long anonymous article in the *Edinburgh Medical and Surgical Journal*, 1820, 16: 481–509 on 'The present state of the profession of physic in England' in which it was said that the present system was ridiculous and that the College had 'usurped power' which was 'despotically exercised'.

24. In part this was due to the fact that the universities of Aberdeen and St Andrews had long granted their MDs to English practitioners for a fee of 10 guineas and two letters of recommendation from physicians. This put Scottish MDs in bad odour with the London physicians, who delighted in lumping together all Scottish MDs, regardless of the university, and condemning their 'diplomas' as useless bits of paper which could be purchased by anyone without test or examination or even setting foot in Scotland.

25. James Fernandez Clarke, *Autobiographical Recollections*, London, 1874, p. 67.

26. ibid., p. 67.

27. ibid., p. 68.

28. ibid., p. 69. See also Samuel Squire Sprigge's outstanding biography of Wakley. *The Lancet*'s abrasiveness seems to have diminished when he became an MP and a Coroner. Although radical in the House of Commons he was much less virulent than he had been as editor of his journal – and much more effective as a consequence.

29. Several papers from the *Medico-Chirurgical Transactions*, 1832, vol. 17 are reported at length in the *Medical and Physical Journal*, 1833, 69: 34–63, but the paper by Hodgkin, 'On some morbid appearances of the absorbent glands and spleen', was not one of them, and was saved for 'private perusal'. They missed that one.

30. The internationalism of the *Edinburgh Medical and Surgical Journal* no doubt reflected the origin of Edinburgh graduates. From 1781–1826 out of 2791 Edinburgh MDs, 848 came from Ireland, 819 from Scotland, 706 from England; 225 came from the colonies, 193 were foreigners, *Edinburgh Medical and Surgical Journal*, 1827, 27: 368. Many Edinburgh graduates later practised abroad. In the first half of the nineteenth century the journal contained many papers from East

India Company and Army medical officers, from Europe, West Africa and the Americas.

31. I. Loudon, *Medical Care and the General Practitioner*, Oxford: OUP, 1986.

32. The contents were interesting for their breadth: original communications, foreign medical literature, analytical reviews, medical intelligence (including short obituaries), prices of pharmaceutical products, bills of mortality, medical and meteorological reports, and a monthly catalogue of books on medicine and natural history. It was edited initially by George Man Burrows (see note 36 below), William Royston and Anthony Todd Thomson, all well-known London general practitioners.

33. E. Harrison, *Remarks on the ineffective State of the Practice of Physic in Great Britain*, London, 1806, and *An address to the Lincolnshire Benevolent Medical Society*, London, 1810.

34. G.M. Burrows, *A Statement of Circumstances connected with the Apothecaries Act and its Administration*, London, 1817.

35. The meetings and subsequent developments are reported most fully in the *Medical and Physical Journal* and the *London Medical, Surgical and Pharmaceutical Repository*.

36. There are numerous instances. One will do. Thomas West, surgeon–apothecary of Abingdon in Berkshire, published in 1815 a brief but vivid account of an outbreak of puerperal fever and erysipelas which closely resembled the famous account of Alexander Gordon of Aberdeen. Both accounts are of great historical importance but West's would probably never have been published had there not been a medical periodical suitable for the purpose. See T. West, 'Observations on some diseases, particularly puerperal fever, which occurred in Abingdon and its vicinity in 1813 and 1814', *London Medical Repository*, 1815, 2: 103–5.

37. The notable exceptions are the *Report of the Select Committee on Medical Education*, PP 1834 (602, parts I, II and III) XIII, said to have been of great importance to George Eliot in writing *Middlemarch*; and the disappointingly dull *Reports of the Select Committee on Medical Registration* PP 1847 (620) IX and PP 1847–8 (210 and 702), XV.

4

Medicine and the Victorian scientific press

W.H. Brock

> With a great effort she gave her mind to her Roscoe, reflecting, for the fiftieth time, what an easy subject Chemistry would be if there were no such thing as carbon.
>
> Graham Travers (=Margaret Todd, MD, *Growth. A novel*, 1906, p.98)

It comes as no surprise that a turn-of-the-century medical student, albeit female rather than male, should be obliged to learn chemistry. The long-established iatrochemical tradition dating back to the sixteenth century had long ensured that doctors valued chemistry; indeed, in the eighteenth and early nineteenth centuries many of the more important chemical innovations and discoveries came from practising doctors. It would be merely to state the obvious, therefore, to say that, on the whole, Victorian doctors knew some chemistry and that the keener of them followed its progress. Perusal of the *British Medical Journal* and *The Lancet* especially supports this unsurprising generalization which might easily be extended to doctors' interests in the other 'collateral sciences'[1] of biology and physics. We can go further and state that, other things being equal, the medical profession was the best educated potential audience for the scientific community to address and that its general periodicals and annuals (such as *The Medical Annual*) reflected an expectation that doctors were interested in the general progress of science and keen to hear of its latest developments.

But what of the converse? How much of contemporary medicine did the Victorian scientist know? Or, put another way, how far did Victorian science periodicals reflect medical progress and events? In the second part of this paper I shall present evidence that, far from being a reciprocal phenomenon, the presentation of medical news in the scientific press was sparse and unimpressive. But first, some general points concerning the nineteenth-century scientific press should be made.

The nineteenth-century science periodical

An examination of *The Waterloo Directory of Victorian Periodicals*,[2] a partial list of roughly 29,000 periodicals and newspapers published in Great Britain between 1824 and 1900, suggests that just over 1 per cent (345) of all Victorian science periodicals were issued commercially, as opposed to just over 0.5 per cent (190) that were sponsored by scientific societies and academies. In other words, of the 535 British science periodicals listed by *The Waterloo Directory*, 64 per cent were commercial publications, that is, 1.75 times more than sponsored ones. Although they were not necessarily all equally important for scientific communications or the progress of science, the main growth factor in nineteenth-century science periodicals was undoubtedly a commercial spirit, not the proliferation of specialized societies.

This flourishing of commercial science, from five general science journals in 1815 to more than eighty in 1895,[3] has only recently attracted the attention of historians of science and specialists in Victorian periodicals.[4] Probably because they have usually been concerned with the origins of scientific periodicals in the seventeenth century, historians of science and science librarians have implied that science journals – with honourable exceptions like *The Philosophical Magazine* and *Nature* (f.1869) – have been society-sponsored. The overwhelming significance of commercial journals during the Victorian era has thereby been overlooked.

Commercial journals served a set of important functions for the scientific community. They speeded up publication at times when the proceedings of scientific societies appeared only intermittently or twice a year; they provided intelligence of science in foreign journals for those who had no access to large libraries; they aired controversies and allowed the issues to be resolved promptly; they accepted for publication the minor, and sometimes trivial, research with which learned societies could not be bothered; they continued to cater for popular 'amateur' science when science was undergoing the rigour of specialization; and they provided a platform for 'alternative sciences' by accepting for publication original findings and speculations that were considered unorthodox by the ruling cliques of learned societies.[5]

Three kinds of commercial science journal may be distinguished: those launched by the proprietors as purely financial speculations, to be abandoned immediately their profitability became questionable; those launched altruistically by their owners for the good of science, and supported by the unpaid contributions of readers, the journal being heavily subsidized until either it was solvent or the owner approached bankruptcy; and those launched with a genuine desire to further science and to give proprietor, editor and possibly contributors a fair financial return for their time and efforts.[6] Such journals may also be classified into subject categories: periodicals that attempted to cover the spectrum of the sciences, specialized journals of chemistry, physics, botany, etc., general journals which stood 'between the High Priests of pure science and the humble votaries who would know its wisdom',[7] periodicals for the upper- and middle-class amateur and tyro, and those whose readership was drawn from the working-class artisan and mechanic.

Although there were more commercial than society-sponsored science journals founded during the nineteenth century, few of them had long lives. Indeed, whereas perhaps the majority of society-sponsored journals have survived in one form or another into the 1990s, of the commercial journals founded before 1900, scarcely a dozen – *Phil.Mag.* (1798), *The Lancet* (1823), *Magazine of Natural History* (1828, now *Journal of Natural History*), *Geological Magazine* (1858), *Chemist and Druggist* (1859), *Engineering* (1866), *The Practitioner* (1868), *Nature* (1869), *Observatory* (1877), *Annals of Botany* (1887) and *Science Progress* (1894) – are still published. Here lies another reason for the neglect of those that fell victim to market forces. Learned societies have a captive audience of members and specialized libraries for whom fluctuating subscription rates have had little effect until recent years. Provided their printing and postage bills were covered, societies were not over-concerned with profitability. Commercial journals were; and were at the mercy of the financial solvency, as well as the personal whims, of proprietors and publishing houses, the changing tastes of their readers and advertisers and the general economic climate.[8]

In 1824 a *Blackwood's Magazine* contributor, William Stevenson, presented a strong case for a reciprocal influence between periodical publications and the intellectual progress of the nation. 'Periodical publications', he wrote, 'are a surer index of the state of progress of the mind, than works of a higher character.'[9] How did the burgeoning scientific communities – the separate but overlapping communities of cultivators, practitioners and researchers of nature[10] – fit into the rapidly changing world of Georgian and early Victorian Britain? What light can scientific periodicals throw upon this changing world – a world in which, in Tennyson's later words, the changeless law was change itself?[11]

British science between 1820 and 1850 has been characterized in many different ways: the heroic–biographical; the thematic–philosophical and the institutional–sociological, but periodicals have rarely been used in these delineations. Although Alfred Russel Wallace, in *The Wonderful Century*, took the Dickensian view that the nineteenth century had been one of the scientific 'best of times–worst of times', the interpretation to which most of us remain indebted as teachers is the intellectual and philosophical one which the Victorian 'Venerable Bede', John Theodore Merz, fashioned in his encyclopaedic *History of European Thought in the Nineteenth Century*. This was a scientific version of Mark Pattison's 'Tendencies of Religious Thought' in *Essays and Reviews* or Leslie Stephen's *History of English Thought in the Eighteenth Century*. Like these earlier religious and philosophical models, Merz's *History of European Thought* was unconcerned with social history.[12] Merz neglected technology, the individual innovators themselves, and the institutions, including periodicals, that historians of science now find so significant. Instead, in his typology, astronomical, atomic, kinetic, physical, morphological, genetic, vitalistic, psycho-physical and statistical views (corresponding, of course, to astronomy, chemistry, electromagnetic theory, thermo-dynamics, natural history, evolution, physiology and genetics, psychology and probability theory) were seen as elements in the cultural spirit of the competing nations of France, Germany and Britain.

A less cumbersome and complicated, but still basically Merzian, approach is that attempted by Harold Sharlin in *The*

Convergent Century.[13] Here Victorian science is epitomized as a search for unification, synthesis and simplification, which is triumphantly realized. Thus Faraday in 1833 demonstrates that all five known forms of electricity (frictional, voltaic, magneto, thermo and animal) are identical qualitatively and quantitatively; Faraday, again, establishes parallels between electric magnetic phenomena; Fresnel and the British School of Mathematical Physics argue for the greater simplicity of the wave theory of light over the emission theory, a view which in turn enables Maxwell to make the unification between electromagnetism and light, which in turn is paralleled by the collapse of other imponderable bodies into thermodynamics; meanwhile further unifications are sought by chemists through the atomic theory, Prout's reduction of the elements to one matter and the use of analogies from inorganic to the organic domain; finally the geologists, biologists and astronomers converge upon the theory of evolution.

Convergence, simplification, unification, quantification are, indeed, all characteristics of British science in the nineteenth century; though historians need also to probe the well-springs of this search for simple invariance amidst the changing complexity of nature. In Faraday's case, for example, as L. P. Williams says, they came from the 'deepest intuitions about the physical word [which] sprang from his religious faith in the Divine origin of Nature'.[14]

More recently historiography has rejected the assumption that the 'motive for scientific work is merely the spirit of free inquiry'.[15] In the case of Victorian science, the characterization must therefore now also embrace an investigation of 'the relation between the practice and the social place of physical scientists . . . [and] to examine the way in which the knowledge of physical nature has been produced, marketed and consumed'.[16] For example, Geoffrey Cantor, in his *Optics after Newton*, portrays the introduction of the wave theory of light in the 1830s in terms of scientific politics and method and as a catalyst for the scientific reconstruction of British science. Again, in several places, J.B. Morrell has evoked portraits of British science in the 1820s and 1830s by 'using a schematic typology based on function, location and social class', while he and Arnold Thackray have brilliantly examined the origins and development of one particular institution – the British Association for the Advancement of Science – entirely in terms of its members, their interests and the coteries of 'gentlemen' who formed the

Association's management committees.[17] Although periodicals were never a principal tool of their studies, Cantor, Morrell and Thackray all make good use of them in their narratives.

Perhaps we can go further with periodicals, bearing in mind Stevenson's observation that they are measures of the intellectual state of a society. Suppose we select an arbitrary year, 1824, and examine what is characteristic about both the available science journals and the science itself as reflected in the pages of such agents of primary communication.[18] On the one hand there were available the journals of the London scientific élite societies – the Royal Society's *Transactions*, as well as those of the Linnean and Geological Societies, the *Memoirs* of the Royal Astronomical Society,[19] and the Royal Institution's *Quarterly Journal of Science* under the quirky editorship of Thomas Brande,[20] with its strong bias towards medical and pharmaceutical chemistry – and, at Cambridge, the *Transactions* of the Philosophical Society where the bulk of British mathematical papers found a home at this time.

On the other hand, there was already a surprisingly large group of commercial journals, including the new weekly *The Lancet* with which Thomas Wakley pricked the wen of contemporary medical practice, the monthly *Philosophical Magazine* (printed and co-edited by Richard Tayor), its principal London rival, Richard Phillips' *Annals of Philosophy*, and from the Edinburgh presses, the competitive duo of Robert Jameson's *Edinburgh New Philosophical Journal* and its rival the *Edinburgh Journal of Science* edited by David Brewster.[21] In addition, at a lower level of sophistication, there were several monthly patent magazines, including *The Repertory of Arts*, Newton's *London Journal of Arts and Sciences* and Gill's *Technical Repository*. Finally, to complete the picture, there were the new artisan journals: *The Mechanic's Magazine*, *The London Mechanics' Register*, *The Mechanics' Weekly Journal*, *The Chemist* and *The Mechanics' Oracle*. This list of journals is not exhaustive (Thomas Bell's *Zoological Journal* was first launched in 1824, for example) but, catering as they did for all shapes and sizes of scientific concern, they are a clear indicator of the strength of interest in science/technology in the 1820s. Nor should we overlook the existence of the heavy monthlies and quarterlies – though, unusually, in this particular year of 1824, out of the 208 essays published in the *Quarterly Review*, the *Edinburgh Review* and *Blackwood's Magazine*, only two were explicitly concerned with scientific matters.[22]

By 1824, however, as Stevenson noted,[23] a division of labour had taken place when 'it was found that almost every one department [of the general magazines of the 1800s] was sufficient to support and sell its own peculiar magazine'. Not surprisingly, then, proprietors of existing journals and entrepreneurs who saw clearly the cash value of Koenig's mechanized press for producing rapid and large press runs looked at the equation between 'intellect' and the huge populations of urban labouring men. In London, the ex-naval officer and economist, Thomas Hodgkin, together with the Scots patent agent, John Robertson, launched the *Mechanics' Magazine* in August 1823 for 'the diffusion of useful information'. Six months later, in April 1824, Hodgkin began *The Chemist* for practical men. Not to be outdone, in July, Alexander Tilloch, the ageing owner and editor of the *Philosophical Magazine* (whose printer, Taylor, had been a patentee of the mechanized press), began *The Mechanics' Oracle* for 'the instruction and improvement of the working classes'.

In practice, Tilloch's journal was far too lavishly illustrated to be sold cheaply, and at 8 pence a week it proved too expensive to capture high sales. Hodgkin's *Chemist* also went the way of all flesh after eleven months of publication, leaving Robertson's *Mechanics' Magazine* (Hodgkin and he fell out after only a few weeks' joint editorship) as the leader in this class market and a model for both other rival mechanics' magazines and for Chambers' *Edinburgh Journal* of 1832 and Charles Knight's *Penny Magazine* of the same year.

If historians have universally drawn attention to the proliferation of specialized scientific societies as characteristic of the Victorian period, what I am drawing attention to here again is the even greater proliferation of commercial journals of primary and secondary communication. This 'golden stream' has still to be properly charted.[24] However, there is a distinctive feature of this proliferation which points to another characteristic of early Victorian science.

In her doctoral thesis, Susan Sheets-Pyenson has appropriately labelled the cultural diffusion journals like *Mechanics' Magazine* as exemplifying 'low science' as opposed to the 'high science' of the gentlemen scientists of the metropolitan learned societies. 'Low science' was not solely dependent for its sustenance on 'high science' (i.e. it was not just popular science), but was a worker's science with its 'own canons of scientific investigation, criticism and explanation'[25] – canons which stressed the roles of experience, the practical and the applied, and which explicitly maintained that science/technology was for all and was not just the privilege of gentlemen scientists. Since it was an area of knowledge which anyone, however humble, could understand and generate for themselves, not surprisingly there was a strong emphasis upon mechanical inventions and improvements, and, as David Allen has excitingly shown, on natural history.[26]

Now, apart from men like George Birkbeck and Henry Brougham, who partially bridged the gap between high and low science and their respective journals, the gentlemen of science largely ignored the existence of this huge reservoir of low science. As the century progressed, of course, the gulf between low and high science was closed as educational machinery from the Department of Science and Art built bridges from high science, while the heir to the *Mechanics' Magazine* – the *English Mechanic* (f.1865) – constructed scaffolding from below. High science itself also characteristically experienced these class divisions, as well as radicalization and campaigns for democratization, as has been brilliantly charted for the Royal Society by Miller and MacLeod, and by Adrian Desmond for medicine and comparative anatomy.[27] Another major journal for bridging the gap was *The Chemical News.*

Medicine in the scientific press

The Chemical News (1859–1932) was the successor of various rival and short-lived journals of chemistry and pharmacy entitled *The Chemist* (1840–58), *Annals of Chymistry and Pharmacy* (1842–43), *Pharmaceutical Times* (1846–49) and *Chemical Gazette* (1842–58), to which may be added the long-lasting official journal of the Pharmaceutical Society, the *Pharmaceutical Journal.* The editor of *The Chemical News,* William Crookes, included in its pages reports of toxicology, materia medica and pharmacy, saying that these features were specifically aimed at the medical reader.[28] In practice, this meant that in the 1860s and 1870s Crookes encouraged lively discussions on food adulteration and the passage of the Public Health Act of 1875. Weekly issues were also filled with articles and lively controversy concerning the cattle plague, water analysis and the disposal of town sewage, in all of which Crookes took a strong personal interest. However, judging from Crookes's adverse comments on the proposed Medical Act being discussed in 1863, which would have placed retail pharmacists under the control of the General Medical Council, he knew his 'medical' readers were chemists and druggists rather than physicians and surgeons.

> We do not suppose that any of our readers have paid much attention to medical politics. The subject is not an inviting one, nor is the study of it in any sense profitable, and we should owe an apology for introducing it now were it not that the interests of a large section of our readers are likely to be placed in some danger.[29]

And he happily reprinted a derogatory note on the General Medical Council from the *Pall Mall Gazette* in 1866 which emphasized the high costs of its deliberations.[30]

'Having so persistently regretted the ignorance of chemistry which is prevalent amongst our medical men', Crookes warmly welcomed Thudichum's specialized journal, *Annals of Chemical Medicine*, which first appeared in 1880.[31] He also noted James Simpson's hopes and expectations concerning the future possibilities of pharmacy,[32] and he gave fulsome space to one of Hofmann's evening lectures, given in 1861 for the Committee of Council on Education. In this important lecture, on the reasons for studying chemistry, Hofmann had highlighted the message that organic chemistry would revolutionize therapeutics:

> Medicine some years ago found itself in a predicament very similar to that of agriculture at the same period; its resources appeared to be in a state of exhaustion, the rich capital of facts accumulated in the department of organic morphology by the industry of the anatomist, and by the acumen of the physiologist, could not yield its full fruits until an equivalent of knowledge had been drawn from the study of bio-chemical phenomena.[33]

But now, Hofmann (echoing Liebig) suggested, that the age of vitalism had passed, chemical analysis would unlock medicine's remaining mysteries. Even so, by the 1880s it is difficult to find anything in the journal relating to medicine.

Founded in 1798, the *Philosophical Magazine* quickly established a reputation for its eclectic coverage of the sciences. In fact, however, its reportage of medicine was never outstanding, being about 12 per cent of its contents, or between four and eight articles out of the seventy or so published in the six months that made up each volume. After 1818 there was barely one medical contribution a year, and by the 1860s even the occasional article had disappeared as the journal assumed a more specialized physics and chemistry identity. As to the medical subjects its first editor, Alexander Tilloch, was willing to publish in the period 1800 to 1820, they fell almost exclusively into five categories. There were regular articles on Jenner's cowpox inoculation (upon which Dr Robert John Thornton was a regular correspondent); contributions on disinfection and fumigation as practised by the French and in particular the work on chlorine fumigation conducted by Guyton de Morveau; and reports of surgical cases treated by John Taunton at the Finsbury Dispensary, with implied support for the charity, the London Truss Society. (Taunton was probably a friend of Tilloch's and, through him, of Richard Taylor, Tilloch's editorial successor; Taylor's son, William Francis, was to marry Taunton's grand-daughter.) Not surprisingly, in the period 1814 to 1816, when Spurzheim was touring Britain, phrenology also attracted a good deal of attention from medical contributors. A final category of medical interest consisted of reprints or abstracts of papers published by the Animal Chemistry Club in the Royal Society's *Transactions*. Allen and Pepys' experimental work on respiration in 1809 also fell into this category.[34]

That surgeons and general practitioners were expected to form part of Tilloch's potential readership seems clear from his publication in 1810 of an anonymous suggestion for improving surgical instruments through developing analogies with carpenters' tools. Occasionally readers addressed medical queries. In 1817, for example, a 72-year-old anonymous patient who had 'lately seen some useful medical papers in *Philosophical Magazine* . . . in which medical knowledge of the first importance has been communicated to the public', offered a reward of fifty guineas for the cure of his ailments.[35] These included the death-toll symptoms of gallstones, jaundice, 'hernia humoralis', a disordered stomach, flatulence and flocculant gassy urine!

If the medical content of *Philosophical Magazine* reached its nadir in the 1820s, one might expect that, because medical men were usually well-represented in their memberships, medical lectures would have been prominent in the programmes of Literary and Philosophical Societies, and hence in their published proceedings. However, to judge from the *Proceedings of the Royal Institution*, this was by no means the case. In the seventeen thick volumes of the latter from 1851 to 1904, only eighteen articles have a medical orientation. Admittedly, these do reflect important current concerns within both the scientific and medical communities: John Conolly on the treatment of insanity in 1854; Robert Druitt on the design of houses in relation to health in 1858; John H. Bridges on civilization, health and the infant mortality rate in 1867; John Tyndall's Pasteurian essays on dust and disease in the decade 1867 to 1877; Alfred H. Garrod on the sphygmograph in 1874 (curiously one of the very few articles in Victorian general scientific literature on the enormously important development of medical diagnostic instrumentation); Victor Horsley on hydrophobia, the topic of the day in 1891, and on the destructive effects of projectiles on (animal) brain tissue in 1894; and an interesting group of bacteriological articles in the 1880s from Edward E. Klein (of vivisection notoriety) on scarlet fever and other infectious diseases, and by G. Sims Woodhead on diphtheria antitoxin treatment in 1895.[36]

One particularly interesting lecture was given in May 1860 by the President of the Royal College of Physicians, Thomas Mayo, 'on the relations of the public to the science and practice of medicine'.[37] Mayo noted the inbuilt tension between client and practitioner, the one in pain and annoyed at having to apply for help, the other intellectually and emotionally involved in treatment. Cooperation between doctor and patient was essential if success was to be achieved; and this was only possible if a well-informed public made sensible choices 'between conflicting schools of medicine'.[38] Thus, whereas the medical profession had tried, and speedily dropped, a cold-water treatment of fever introduced by Drs Currie and Wright of Liverpool in the 1820s, a poorly informed public had eagerly taken up the hydrotherapy of 'an untutored Silesian peasant' (Priessnitz). Since 1842, in the wake of Liebig's demonstration of the role of oxygen in human metabolism, the action of the skin in hydrotherapy had become better understood. Mayo quoted the warning of Liebig's pupil, Henry Bence Jones, that death could ensue from the over-zealous promotion of oxidation in hydrotherapy as an example of the 'expediency of an increased amount of medical and physiological knowledge of the public, who select for themselves both medical systems and medical advisers'.[39] Conversely, doctors had a duty towards patients of reducing cases to general laws by using their powers of imagination, memory and speculation. This gave Mayo another opportunity to chastise what he considered unorthodox, this time homoeopathy. But it also gave him the chance to argue against specialism in medicine which he viewed as encouraged by the public's expectation of an individual doctor's bent 'in favour of some one group of cases and diseases'. Obviously annoyed by the pretensions of some alienists (although mental disease was an area for which Mayo was well known), he warned that:

> The public prevents those medical practitioners, who have gained reputation in this speciality from becoming acquainted with other coterminous disease by excluding them from attendance on other diseases; and thus necessarily diminishes their power of diagnosis of mental disease *itself.* Hence arises ignorance of practitioners both in certifying the presence of insanity, and in giving evidence on it in courts of justice.[40]

Finally, although the moral and social education of doctors was now well handled, Mayo claimed, the public still too frequently neglected its moral duty towards new practitioners insofar as, despite frequently possessing a superior general education to their patients or their families, their position in society was 'one of comparative exclusion'.[41]

If Mayo's address rode several hobby-horses of orthodox medicine, it remained a rare example of a medical man urging an 'increased acquaintance on the part of the public with medical and physiological principles'.

Although medicine was never a regular annual feature of the Royal Institution's Friday Evening Discourses, over a lifetime's membership of the Royal Institution during the second half of the nineteenth century an RI member would have had a fair impression of the contributions that contemporary medicine was making to public health. He or she would have been particularly aware of the transformation from a miasmatic to a germ theory approach towards disease, but would have learned nothing of anaesthesia, pharmacology or clinical medicine.

A less uneven tradition of 'state of the art' review was to become a particular feature of the quarterly *Science Progess* (7 vols 1894–98) after its re-establishment by N. H. Alcock and W. G. Freeman in 1906. The new developments in biochemistry, as well as nuclear physics, were to prove particularly valuable in the period up to 1920. In this the editors reflected the aspirations of the journal's founding editors, Henry C. Burdett (its financier) and the botanist, J. Bretland Farmer, who hoped 'to obviate the bane of excessive specialization'.[42]

What then of the weekly journal *Nature* which, under the founding editorship of the astronomer Norman Lockyer and the financial support of its publisher Alexander Macmillan, gradually became essential reading for the British (and increasingly an overseas) professionally qualified scientific audience?[43] Although Lockyer never made any explicit policy statement, he clearly did not feel there was a large medical readership to be gained for *Nature* or wooed from its weekly *Lancet* or *BMJ*. Consequently, *Nature* did not report medical matters to any great degree or review medical texts. Like *Philosophical Magazine* earlier, and *Proceedings of the Royal Institution* contemporaneously, it was content to reflect medical issues which closely pertained to scientific matters or to the health of the nation. Thus, although Lockyer strongly supported the 1870s movement for the higher education of women, *Nature* virtually ignored the Edinburgh University scandal of matriculated women being refused their medical degrees.[44] On the other hand, *Nature* strongly supported and reported the new experimental physiology and defended vivisection during the debates of the 1880s. It also regularly included editorials and articles on matters concerned with sewage disposal, the germ theory (including reports for and against Henry Charlton Bastian's anomalous results over spontaneous generation). A series of reports by S. Stricker on British and German medical education in 1870 was followed by others advocating the teaching of the principles of state medicine to medical students, and periodic reportage of changes in the medical curriculum and examination system.[45] Lockyer's policy on public health was clearly that of his principal contributor on the subject, Edwin Lankester. The latter, in a November 1870 article on the current scarlet fever epidemic, gave advice on how families should deploy disinfectants and concluded:

> I am convinced that the holocaust of victims that we annually offer to this Moloch of scarlet fever arises from ignorance, and that a general knowledge alone of the facts stated . . . can suffice to drive from us this plague, so disgraceful alike to our intelligence and our humanity.[46]

Perhaps the best-known, and only, abortive attempt to provide specific medical information in a popular science journal in the nineteenth century is that of the *English Mechanic.* Primarily devoted to technical issues in carpentry and metalwork, combined with informative articles and queries on astronomy, chemistry, electricity and microscopy, *English Mechanic* had largely ignored medical matters, until 1873. In 1870 it reported how 2000 doctors [*sic*] had attended a meeting at the Royal Polytechnical Institute in Regent's Street to witness a trial 'of a new mode of conveying practical instructions in a department of surgery' given by Dr Balmanno Squire. But the journal's interest here was really in the technique whereby Squire threw magnified images of a patient's anatomy on to a huge screen.[47] Similarly, *English Mechanic*'s perennial interest in galvanism and medical electricity emphasized the building of an electric coil rather than a prophylactic technique. As in the other journals surveyed, however, the periodical gave publicity in the 1870s to new ideas about germs, it gave advice on disinfectants, and warned readers of the mortal dangers of arsenic in coloured wallpapers.

One of the *English Mechanic*'s occasional medical correspondents was Dr William Henry Stone (1830–91), a lecturer in materia medica and physics at St.Thomas's Hospital where he specialized in electrotherapy.[48] On 18 July 1873 Stone began a weekly, signed, medical question and answer column. Clearly aware that colleagues might be critical, he carefully laid down the parameters of what the column would and would not attempt to do. No doubt because *English Mechanic* readers were often controversial and unorthodox in their views, Stone refused to discuss rival theories of medicine:

> Without expressing an opinion on 'acid cures', 'hydropathy', botany or homeopathy, I may say at once their very magnitude, either for good or evil, excludes them. They are best left to learned societies, to systematic treatises, and to the general voice of society.[49]

Nor was the column to be a shop 'for feeble and perfunctory medical advice'. Still less was it to be:

> for the incautious hawking about of recipes which, though one man's food, may be another man's poison. To a querist who sought advice, I could go thus far: I could say whether the symptoms named bore a grave or trivial interpretation; I could even, at times, guide him in the proper way for obtaining sound and trustworthy advisers. More than this I feel sure he could not reasonably expect.

Stone saw his column as standing 'intermediate between the professional and the non-professional world'. Like Edwin Lankester in *Nature* he saw the column as an opportunity to purvey information and advice on sanitary matters rather than on medicine *per se*.

> It could give hints about dress, food, hours of work and play, and facts about climate and emigration; suggestions for the prevention of diseases to which artisans are especially liable; it might discuss symptoms of warming and ventilation; and even venture upon guidance in the commoner and less severe emergencies which admit of domestic treatment.[50]

Following this announcement of his editorial policy, Stone launched an attack on 'the ugly absurdity' of stays and their relation to problems of indigestion.

To a modern reader Stone's advice column appears innocuous, proffering sound domestic advice on precautions to take during the outbreak of typhoid fever in August 1872 and offering sympathy to victims of consumption. However, violent attacks on him in *The Lancet* and *British Medical Journal* and accusations that he was offering a free medical service forced Stone, with the concurrence of the *English Mechanic*'s editor, John Passmore Edwards, to abandon the column after only thirteen weeks.[51] Insofar as other established scientists who wrote for the paper, such as Richard Proctor and Andrew Noble, usually wrote pseudonymously or anonymously, Stone's mistake was surely to publish his name. His career did not suffer, since he went on to become a Harveian Lecturer in 1887, but *English Mechanic*, which folded in 1926, never again attempted to provide medical articles.

Stone's experience forms a fitting end to this inquiry. It is clear that medicine did not figure prominently in the periodical literature to which the non-medical community contributed and read. Even the Royal Society, which continued to have a large percentage of medically qualified Fellows throughout the Victorian period, shunned overt medical and surgical papers in the *Proceedings* and *Transactions*, and confined itself to anatomical and physiological papers.[52] Given the phenomenal growth of the powerful and specialized medical press, which other contributors to this volume have considered, the low profile of medicine in specialized and general journals of science is scarcely surprising. Clearly, in the commercial sphere, proprietors who owned one or several science journals preferred not to mix scientific and medical titles, while, within their general science journals, medical articles and news seem to have been largely confined to issues of public health or to matters pertaining to medicine and its collateral sciences of physiology, chemistry and pharmacy. Nor were the annual reviews of the progress of science, such as John Timbs's *Year-Book of Facts in Science and Art* (1838–80) or the American *Annual of Scientific Discovery* (1850–79), any different.[53] Neither included medical events in their compilations, unlike Louis Figuier's *L'année scientifique et industrielle* which explicitly addressed 'public health, physiology and medicine'.[54] The contrast with the *Medical Annual* which, under the editorship of John Taylor (who also edited *Science Gossip*), regularly reported the year's developments in chemistry, astronomy, physics and biology to its medical audience (or with William Braithwaite's *The Retrospect of Medicine*) is stark.[55] From the evidence of periodicals it is hard to resist the conclusion that Victorian medical men were likely to be better informed about science than their scientific colleagues were about medicine.

Notes

1. N.G. Coley, 'The collateral sciences in the work of Golding Bird (1814–1854)', *Med.Hist.* 1969, 13: 363–76.

2. M. Wolff, J.S. North, D. Dearing, eds, *The Waterloo Directory of Victorian Periodicals*, Waterloo, Ont.: University of Waterloo, 1977.

3. C. Mitchell, ed., *Newspaper Press Directory*, annual from 1846. See volume for 1895.

4. A.J. Meadows, *Communication in Science*, London, Butterworth, 1974, ch. 3; R.M. Gascoigne, *A Historical Catalogue of Scientific Periodicals 1665–1900*, New York, Greenwood, 1985.

5. S. Lilley, 'Nicholson's Journal (1797–1813)', *Annals of Science*, 1948–50, 6: 78–101.

6. J.C. Loudon, *Magazine of Natural History*, 1830, 3: Preface.

7. *Science Gossip*, 1865, 1: Preface.

8. The previous five paragraphs are drawn from W.H. Brock, 'The development of commercial science journals in Victorian Britain' in A.J. Meadows, ed., *Development of Science Publishing in Europe*, Amsterdam: Elsevier, 1980, 95–122. This examines *Phil.Mag.*, *The Laboratory* and *English Mechanic*.

9. [W. Stevenson], 'On the reciprocal influence of the periodical publications and the intellectual progress of this century', *Blackwood's Magazine*, 1824, 16: 518–28. Although promised, the essay was not continued.

10. N. Reingold, 'Definitions and speculations: the professionalization of science in America in the nineteenth century' in A. Oleson and S.C. Brown, eds, *The Pursuit of Knowledge in the Early American Republic*, Baltimore and London, Johns Hopkins University Press, 1976, 33–69.

11. *De Profundis*, 1880.

12. J.T. Merz, *A History of European Thought in the Nineteenth Century*, 4 vols, Edinburgh: Blackwood, 1904–12; reprint Dover, New York, 1965. Pattison's unfinished essay is in *Essays and Reviews*, London, J. Parker, 1860. L. Stephen, *History of English Thought in the Eighteenth Century*, 2 vols, London, Smith Elder, 1881.

13. H.J. Sharlin, *The Convergent Century*, London and New York, 1966. Note also Susan F. Cannon, *Science in Culture: the Early Victorian Period*, New York, Science History Publications, 1978.

14. L.P. Williams, *Michael Faraday*, London, Chapman and Hall, 1965, 102–6.

15. S. Schaffer, 'History of physical sciences' in P. Corsi and P. Weindling, eds, *Information Sources in the History of Science and Medicine*, London and Boston, 1983, p. 287.

16. ibid, p. 286.

17. G. Cantor, *Optics after Newton*, Manchester: Manchester University Press, 1983; J.B. Morrell, 'Individualism and the structure of British science in 1830', *Hist.Stud.Phys.Sci.*, 1971, 3: 183–204; J.B. Morrell and A. Thackray, *Gentlemen of Science*, Oxford, Clarendon Press, 1981.

18. Brock, op. cit. (8) and W.H. Brock and A.J. Meadows, *The Lamp of Learning. Taylor & Francis and the Development of Science Publishing*, London: Taylor & Francis, 1984.

19. In 1824, with the exception of the *Phil.Trans.Roy.Soc.*, these journals were all printed by Richard Taylor who, from 1828, also began to print for the Royal Society. By then, however, he had lost the contract with the Royal Astronomical Society. See Brock and Meadows, op. cit. (18).

20. M. Berman, *Social Change and Scientific Organization*, London, 1978, 141–3.

21.W.H. Brock, 'Brewster as a scientific journalist' in A. Morrison-Low and J.R.R. Christie, eds, *David Brewster: Martyr of Science*, Edinburgh, HMSO, 1984.

22. [L. Horner], 'Mineralogical systems', *Edinburgh Review*, 1824, 39: 488–501; [H. Brougham], 'Scientific education of the people', ibid., 1824, 41: 96–122.

23. Stevenson, op. cit. (9), p. 524.

24. M. Wolff, 'Charting the golden stream' in John M. Robson, ed., *Editing Nineteenth-Century Texts*, Toronto, 1967. Note, however, the helpful aid produced by R.M. Gascoigne, *A Historical Catalogue of Scientific Periodicals 1665–1900*, New York: Greenwood, 1985.

25. S. Sheets-Pyenson, 'Popular science periodicals in Paris and London: the emergence of a low scientific culture, 1820–1875', *Ann.Sci.*, 1985, 42: 549–72, based on her *Low Scientific Culture in London and Paris 1820–1875* (unpub.Ph.D. University of Pennsylvania, 1976).

26. D.E. Allen, *The Naturalist in Britain. A Social History*, London, Allen Lane, 1976.

27. D.A. Miller, 'Between hostile camps. Davy's presidency of the Royal Society', *Brit.J.Hist.Sci.*, 1983, 16: 1–48; R.M. MacLeod, 'Whigs and savants: reflections on the reform movement in the Royal Society, 1830–48' in I. Inkster and J.B. Morrell, eds., *Metropolis and Province. Science in British Culture, 1780–1850*, London, 1983; A. Desmond, *The Politics of Evolution*, Chicago: Chicago University Press, 1989.

28. *Chem.News* 1861,3: 1.

29. ibid. 1863, 7: 300 and ibid. 1864, 9: 1.

30. ibid. 1866, 13: 143.

31. ibid. 1880, 40: 10. The *Annals of Chemical Medicine*, which deserves further study, spanned two volumes, 1879–81.

32. *Chem.News* 1868, 18: 82.

33. ibid. 1861, 3: 35. This is possibly the first English use of the Germanic term 'biochemical'.

34. E.g., R.J. Thornton, 'A case of cowpox at Fulwood's Rents', *Phil.Mag.* 1805, 20: 36–59, plus other articles on smallpox, pp. 143-53, 236-55; Anon, 'Report on National Vaccine Establishment for 1814' ibid. 1815, 4: 163–7; M. Bonefus, 'Fumigations with oxygenated muriatic acid', ibid. 1806–7, 26: 71–2; J. Taunton, 'Report of surgical cases at the Finsbury Dispensary', ibid. 1806–7, 26: 253–7; *idem*, 'Case of organic lesion of the brain', ibid. 1810, 35: 59–61; T. Forster, [Reports and articles on phrenology], ibid. 1814, 44: 215–16, 305–12; ibid. 1815, 45: 44–50, 50–63, 129–32; W.B. Brande, 'Effects of magnesia in preventing an increase of uric acid in urine' [Animal Chemistry Club], ibid. 1810, 36: 8–16; W. Allen and J.H. Pepys, ibid. 1809, 34: 379–87.

35. Anon, 'Medical premium', *Phil.Mag.* 1817, 49: 87–90.

36. E.g. J. Conolly, 'On the characters of insanity', *Proc.Roy.Inst.*, 1854, 1: 375–81; R. Druitt, 'On houses in relation to health', ibid. 1859, 3: 133–6; J.H. Bridges, 'On the influence of civilization upon health', ibid. 1869, 5: 470–4; J. Tyndall, 'On dust and disease', ibid. 1870, 6: 6–14; *idem*, 'The optical condition of the atmosphere and its bearings

on putrefaction and infection', ibid. 1876, 8: 6–27; *idem*, 'Researches on the deportment and vital resistance of putrefactive and infective organisms', ibid. 1877, 8: 467–77; A.H. Garrod, 'The heart and the sphygmograph', ibid. 1874, 7: 214–17; V. Horsley, 'Hydrophobia' ibid. 1891, 13: 342–52; *idem*, 'The destructive effects of projectiles', ibid. 1894, 14: 228–38; E. Klein, 'The etiology of scarlet fever', ibid. 1887, 12: 150–8; *idem*, 'Infectious diseases, their nature, cause and mode of spread', ibid. 1891, 13: 277–92; G.S. Woodhead, 'The antitoxic serum treatment of diphtheria', ibid. 1895, 14: 433–50.

37. T. Mayo, 'On the relations of the public to the science and practice of medicine', *Proc.Roy.Inst.* 1860, 3: 258–60.

38. ibid., p. 258.

39. ibid., pp. 259–60.

40. ibid., p. 262.

41. ibid., p. 263.

42. Preface *Science Progress* 1894, 1.

43. On *Nature* see A.J. Meadows, *Science and Controversy. A Biography of Sir Norman Lockyer*, Basingstoke: Macmillan, 1972; and the centenary essays by R.M. MacLeod in *Nature* 1969, 224: 423–72.

44. For brief allusions, see *Nature* 1869–70, 1: 25 and 1871–72, 5: 57–58.

45. S. Stricker, 'The medical schools of England and Germany', *Nature* 1870, 2: 349–50, 369–70; 1870–71, 3: 81–2.

46. E. Lankester, 'The present epidemic of scarlet fever', *Nature* 1870–71, 3: 42.

47. *English Mechanic* 1870, 11: 390.

48. This column has been previously discussed by Charles G. Roland, 'The difficult career of an early medical columnist', *Bull.Med.Lib.Ass.* 1974, 62: 132–6.

49. *English Mechanic* 1873, 17: 457.

50. ibid.

51. 'Popular advice gratis', *Lancet*, ii, 30 August 1873: 310; 'Medical answers to lay correspondents', *BMJ*, ii, 4 October 1873: 403–4; *English Mechanic* 1873, 18: 117, 142.

52. E.g. A.T.H. Waters, 'On the intimate structure, and distribution of the blood vessels of the human lung', *Proc.Roy.Soc.* 1859–60,10: 16–25; R. Boyd, 'Tables of the weights of the human body and the internal organs in the sane and insane of both sexes at various ages', ibid. 1860–62, 11: 124–6; E. Smith, 'On the elimination of urea and urinary water in their relation to the period of the day, season, exertion, food and other influences acting on the cycle of the year', ibid. 1860–62, 11: 204–13.

53. J. Timbs, ed., *The Year-Book of Facts in Science and Art*, London, 1838–1879/80; S. Baird, ed. *Annual of Scientific Discovery*, Boston, 1850–71, then *Annual Record of Science and Industry*, ed. John Trowbridge and Samuel Kneeland, New York, 1872–79. This contained medicine until 1876.

54. L. Figuier, ed., *L'année scientifique et industrelle*, Paris, 1856–1913. This carried a section, 'médecine et physiologie et hygiène publique'.

55. *The Medical Annual and Practitioner's Index*, Bristol, 1883 to date; *The Retrospect of Practical Medicine and Surgery*, London, vols 1–12, 1840–45, then *The Retrospect of Medicine*, 13(1846)–123(1901); cf. Crookes's envious comment on latter, *Chem.News* 1861, 3: 185.

5

'Notorious abominations': architecture and the public health in *The Builder* 1843–83

Ruth Richardson

Victorian interest in health matters, and campaigning journalism in the area of health care, were by no means confined to the pages of the medical press. Advertisements for remedies for every medical complaint festooned newspaper pages. Medical controversies and high-profile campaigns, such as Thomas Wakley's inquests and elections for coroner, gained considerable attention in the popular press.[1] The wider issues of public health and its reform were often raised by Victorian journalists themselves; Mayhew's investigations into the lives of the London poor, published in the *Morning Chronicle*, are a case in point. *Punch* and *Household Words* are two of the many periodicals whose pages served to disseminate the views of public health reformers, as did also the weightier journals, like *Blackwoods* and the *Edinburgh Review*. This paper focuses on the coverage of such issues by the architectural weekly, *The Builder*.

The Builder was founded in 1842 by Joseph Hansom. Hansom is more famous today for his patent safety cab than his journal – perhaps justly so, for *The Builder* was not at first a success and Hansom sold the title to his printers after only twenty-one issues had reached the press. The journal could very easily have become one of the 'infant mortalities' so well described by the Loudons in this volume, had not a young architect by the name of George Godwin been appointed as editor shortly afterwards. Godwin was to serve in that role for the next forty years, and was to establish *The Builder* as the pre-eminent weekly in the field of architecture, construction and sanitary reform.

Bynum and Wilson have commented in this volume: 'without editors, no journals'. Godwin typifies a particular breed of Victorian editor. An autocrat who is said to have been such a workaholic as never to have taken a holiday, his personality was crucial in shaping the journal's tone. His environmental vision and idiosyncratic editorial style gave the journal a voice, and shaped its success. Over his forty years in the post, editor and journal became inseparable in the public mind. As his *Builder* obituary put it: 'he himself . . . really and truly *was* The Builder'.[2]

Godwin was a vigorous, convivial man, contemptuous of humbug and unafraid of confrontation, but more often seeking to improve things through good-heartedness, good information well communicated, and the warm appeal to fellow-feeling. His writings are informative, accurate, honest and earnest and infused with a personality whose enthusiasm and humanity remain contagious even after the passage of a century and more.

Like other editors of his day Godwin was active in professional work and other interests beyond the editorial office. A contemporary observed that he was 'a man behind the scenes in all artistic matters, a leader in many important movements which lay under the surface of affairs, and did not come prominently before the public'.[3] Godwin helped found and was a long-term secretary of the Art Union of London, an organizational dedicated to the wide distribution of art works by subscription lottery.[4] He was a juror for the Great Exhibition of 1851, chaired the committee for the Albert Memorial, and served as District Surveyor for southern Islington for many years. He was also a working architect. During his long and busy life at *The Builder*, he also found time to renovate the church of St Mary Redcliffe in Bristol, to design the villas which surround his interesting church of St Mary Boltons, south of the Old Brompton Road, and – with his brother – to lay out and design much of the Redcliffe estate westwards towards Earls Court.

As was also the case in medicine, nineteenth-century architectural practice was undergoing a process of professionalization, and Godwin both exemplified and aided the process. Although he is not widely known today, he did not go unhonoured in his own era. In 1836 the young Godwin was awarded the Institute of British Architects' first silver medal for an essay on concrete, then an undervalued and underused material. He became a Fellow of the Royal Society. The essay went on to become a standard work of reference for the rest of the century. In later life Godwin, by that time an ex-vice-president, was awarded the RIBA's highest available award. The Royal Gold Medal for 1881 was presented by the Victorian architect G.E. Street for Godwin's lifetime work as a 'literary architect'.[5]

'Literary architect' is a good description. Though trained as an architect, Godwin became a great editor, one whose literary and social interests inform every aspect of his writing. Indeed, it is hardly possible to demarcate between his literary and social thinking. Godwin thought environmentally about practically every aspect of life. For example, *The Builder*'s coverage of the arts includes reviews of theatrical productions, scenery, safe stage lighting, and careful suggestions for adequate fire-proofing and safety exits in theatres, concert halls and other public buildings. Like his close contemporary, Dickens (whom he was later to review, to admire and to know personally), Godwin used his pen to reveal and improve the plight of the inhabitants of the Victorian slum and workhouse.[6]

One of the most resonant of the literary allusions with which Godwin peppered *The Builder*'s pages is to Macaulay's New Zealander. The notion of the Maori who arrives on our shores in centuries to come to excavate the archaeological remains of our own civilization had great appeal for Godwin; after all, we British are said to have been painting ourselves with woad when the Romans invaded, and yet centuries later were capable of appreciatively excavating our old conquerors' remains. The New Zealander emerges in *The Builder*'s pages as a device whereby a longer historical perspective might be applied to contemporary matters: not as in Cobbett's backward-looking appeal to a past golden age, but rather as a prompt to the perception of present-day follies as if through a quizzical future eye.

Godwin believed architecture reflects the state of the civilization which produces it; a belief which caused him to urge that the ruins of our own society should be as beautiful in decay as those of ancient Greece and Rome. He was often roused to real anger by ugly artefacts, bad architecture or shoddy work. In the interests of civilization, he used the journal as a stage for factual, moral, sanitary and aesthetic discussion and instruction, and, when necessary, as a pillory.

By 1848, that year of revolutions across Europe, the journal was well established, and had a growing readership. Its editor recognized, however, that to many unfamiliar with its contents and aims *The Builder* appeared simply as a 'trade paper'. His opening editorial of that year sought to dispel this impression with a discussion of the journal's title, and the following definition later appeared on *The Builder*'s title page:

> The verb 'to build' has been much degraded amongst us, and has lost its full signification. 'Our English word, to build,' says Horne Tooke, 'is the Anglo-Saxon *Byldan*, to confirm, to establish, to make firm and sure and fast, to consolidate, to strengthen; and is applicable to all other things, as well as to dwelling places.'[7]

It is this interest – in 'all other things' – which characterizes *The Builder* during Godwin's long editorship. Title page subtitles indicate the audience he sought to attract. In early numbers Godwin catered for 'The Architect, Engineer, Operative [i.e. the building worker] and Artist', and over the years he added to the list the archaeologist, the art lover and, importantly for us, the sanitary reformer.

Like the history of the cast-iron sewer or the glazed-brick dado, the history of public health seems now to be regarded as quintessentially Victorian, and to our own era the person who appears to embody the character and aims of Victorian public health reform is Edwin Chadwick. A new biographical study has recently appeared, and the centenary of his death has been marked by a timely appeal for a renaissance of public health activity in our own era.[8] Yet the public health movement of the nineteenth century was a movement of many persons, and at least one recent historian has recognized that Chadwick's pre-eminence may have meant that 'others have had less than their due share of credit'.[9] The work of Dr Thomas Southwood Smith in particular deserves revaluation, as do the research and writing of many little-known investigators, several of whom were doctors, who contributed ideas and text to the famous *Sanitary Report*.[10]

George Godwin is another individual whose contribution to the Victorian public health movement has been largely overlooked by posterity. It is time that he too be recognized as the active and effective public health reformer he undoubtedly was. While Chadwick's primary role was in government and administration, Godwin's chosen role was communication and agitation. Even before the publication of Chadwick's *Sanitary Report*, and before Godwin became editor of *The Builder*, Godwin had lobbied the Prime Minister in favour of metropolitan improvements, and had published his views on better architecture for the poor.[11] He was to develop *The Builder* in these and other directions, informing, lobbying and attempting to inspire readers to 'Drain and pave, raise and save'.[12]

In the early days, what we might now consider *sanitary* matters were often referred to in *The Builder* as *sanatory* matters. The spelling of this key word may seem of little moment at this late date, but it may be significant that the older spelling had the wider meaning. The OED defines *sanatory* as 'healing, of or tending to physical or moral health, curative'. *Sanitary*, on the other hand, is defined as 'especially with regard to dirt and infection . . . free from, or designed to obviate influences deleterious to health'. The latter focuses almost entirely upon the physical world, whereas the older usage has what we might term a more holistic approach, encompassing moral as well as physical health. The older spelling is indicative of the Victorian belief that cleanliness was next to godliness, that personal improvement was often contingent upon environmental reform. Our own era may have inverted these concepts, but the concerns remain recognizably similar.

Although appreciated by his contemporaries, and by architectural historians today, Godwin's life's work is less known among historians of medicine. Publication of the forthcoming catalogue and indexes to the entire illustrative output during Godwin's forty years in post, generated by the Builder Project at the University of London, will bring the journal and its editor into greater prominence.[13] Most of the thousands of illustrations are wood engravings of a high standard, commissioned from among the best available talent of the day. *The Builder*'s offices were in Catherine Street, only a stone's throw from the Strand, which was then the hub of the London wood-engraving trade. At one time or another, as our indexes now reveal, Godwin commissioned work from almost every well-known wood engraver in the district.[14]

As one turns the journal's pages, the amplitude of its editor's interests becomes evident. Illustrated articles on country houses new and old, town houses, mansions and palaces, abroad and at home, jostle with others on slum housing, model housing, cellar dwellings, hospital ventilation, new office buildings and warehouses. The latest excavations at Pompeii and Troy are featured alongside railway stations, new sanitary appliances, designs for drains and chimneys, pipes and arches, mosaics, tiles, balustrades and parapets, and ornately carved details from mediaeval cathedral furniture. Ventilation turrets and vaulting make frequent appearance, as do bridges and belfries, fireproofing and damp-proofing, self-acting water closets, reservoirs and reredoses, theatres and mental institutions. Almshouses, lighthouses, workhouses, opera houses, shops and public houses all have their place.

It cannot be doubted that this breadth of coverage affected sales and circulation. During Godwin's forty-year working life at *The Builder*, sales rose and rose; and upon his retirement they fell noticeably.[15]

One has only to consider the enormous public impact and beneficial influence exercised today by the *BMJ* and *The Lancet* to gain some intimation of how important journals must have been in the nineteenth century, when no competition existed from radio or television. Steam applied to paper making, printing and distribution meant that the freshly printed word was available country-wide, even world-wide. When we recall the anticipation of those said to have waited on the New York quay to discover what had happened to Little Nell, we can perhaps imagine the interest, even avidity, with which Victorian periodicals were read.

The Builder's readership spanned the social scale. Professional readership was wide: virtually every Victorian architect of note contributed to the journal's pages at one time or another, and it is clear from its correspondence columns that the journal served as a forum for debate both within the architectural profession and between professions which at this stage were still in process of evolution – architects, engineers, sanitary engineers, structural engineers, and builders of all kinds. Prince Albert kept a well-bound set of the journal. Indeed, Godwin's obituarist in *The Times* ascribed to *The Builder* the inception of Albert's personal interest in sanitary reform.[16] At the other end of society, respectable working-class craft workers certainly valued the journal's contents, for we find a volume of *The Builder* illustrated, alongside vignettes comparing Ancient Rome and Victorian London, on an illuminated trade union membership certificate issued by the Operative Society of Bricklayers of Watford.[17] Even building labourers read, or at least had access to, information in *The Builder*'s pages, for on one occasion Godwin was impelled to publish an apology to several hundreds of them who had reported for work at the site of the new Strand law courts after the journal had published, in good faith, the erroneous news that work was about to begin.[18]

There are difficulties for the historian making the attempt to map or quantify the influence of any periodical. However, indications of *The Builder*'s importance can be gained from the liveliness of the correspondence columns, its increasing volume of advertising, the journal's increasing pagination, and its breadth of readership. Its own pages reveal that relatively early in Godwin's editorship correspondents regarded the journal as influential.[19] As we shall see in a moment, occasions certainly arose in which materials published in *The Builder* were taken up for argument in local and national press, and, indeed, at a parliamentary level.

As for the effectiveness of *The Builder*'s journalism, it can be said that Godwin's labours bore diverse fruit. An editorial published in 1864 arguing for the erection of plaques to preserve and commemorate the surviving homes of great inhabitants, such as Newton, Dryden and Voltaire, met with an immediate response. The Society of Arts (of which Godwin was a Fellow) established a scheme, later adopted by the London County Council, from which developed London's famous blue plaques.[20] The journal instigated and supported campaigns to erect the Shakespeare monument which still stands in Leicester Square, and for a national theatre. The impressive variety of historical and foreign architecture illustrated and intelligently discussed in *The Builder*'s pages probably contributed to the eclecticism of Victorian architecture. Godwin's ideas often had considerable popular appeal. His designation of the ugly South Kensington Museum building as the 'Brompton Boilers' hit a popular nerve. Like Prince Charles's famous 'carbuncle', the name stuck, and public dissatisfaction with its design eventually resulted in the fine new building we know today as the Victoria and Albert Museum.

Godwin's appreciation of good design and the value of craft skills worked its influence upon William Morris and the development of the Arts and Crafts movement. *Builder* coverage also helped create a climate favourable towards saving old buildings from demolition, and other conservation issues. *The Builder* fostered the establishment of the Society for the Preservation of Ancient Buildings, and led the way towards modern listing procedures.[21]

An important aspect of *The Builder*'s influence upon medical history has been analysed by Anthony King, adjusting the historical record concerning the adoption in the second half of the nineteenth century of what have since become familiarly known as 'Nightingale' or 'pavilion' plan hospitals. Tony King has shown that, although the reformed design for hospital layout has often been attributed solely to Miss Nightingale, in reality she was herself perhaps influenced by several major *Builder* editorials published between 1856 and 1858.[22]

The first of these articles opened with a fierce attack on the design of Netley Hospital near Southampton – the first military hospital to be built in England after the Crimea War. The convention of editorial anonymity has done little to assist the accurate attribution of this material. The voice is that of George Godwin, and he himself declared that the views expressed were largely those of John Roberton, a Manchester surgeon. Roberton had studied the transmission of what were then known as 'hospital diseases' and, as a result, he urged that the continental 'pavilion' plan be adopted in this country. He believed the high number of deaths from 'hospital atmosphere' – which seemed to spread such fatal diseases as puerperal fever, septicaemia and erysipelas – could be diminished by the system he had seen in use in France, in which each ward was separated from the next by a garden, with conveniences at one end of each ward and nurses' offices at the other, the wards being cross-ventilated by large windows which stretched from floor to ceiling. Godwin quoted Roberton's recommendations at length and, in his own commentary, pointed out that Gwilt's *Cyclopaedia of Architecture* dated the use of pavilion plan hospitals in France to the eighteenth century. Godwin also considered the practical advantages of other, more recent, European hospitals built along similar lines.

A lively correspondence ensued. Tony King has observed that, between October 1856 and January 1857, comments and correspondence on the matter in *The Builder* 'covered the whole field from the diffusion of gases to the defence of particular ventilation schemes. . . . By June 1857, the Netley designs were being roundly criticized in press and parliament'. The *British Medical Journal* repeated Godwin's assertion that Netley would kill more than it would cure.[23]

The Builder's publication of Roberton's ideas naturally attracted the attention of Florence Nightingale, and Tony King suggests that by the summer of 1857 she and Godwin were in correspondence.[24] Further editorials during the summer and autumn of 1858 attacked the design of most British hospitals, reported upon a tour undertaken by Roberton to the hospitals of twelve major European cities, and laid out desiderata for any future schemes to be erected in the British Isles. Three of these editorials were reprinted by Florence Nightingale as an appendix to her important publication *Notes on Hospitals*, published in 1859, three years after *The Builder*'s first hospital editorials. The same small volume contains her own recommendations for hospital design, which coincide with those of Roberton and Godwin. Although Miss Nightingale surely had independent knowledge of pavilion plan hospital design, it is clear from the fact of her re-publication of *The Builder* editorials that she herself regarded them as the last word on the subject, and not to be improved upon.[25]

The Netley Hospital controversy, initiated and fermented by Roberton, Godwin and Nightingale, resulted in the adoption of pavilion plan designs for virtually all large hospitals, military and civil, erected for a considerable period after these events. Architects who did not adhere to a pavilion layout for hospital building thereafter were defensive about the value of their own designs.[26] The campaign's success had depended crucially upon timing, the power of good information, the repetition of well-informed arguments, lobbying, and the creation of favourable public opinion by the power of the press.

Godwin keenly observed and commented upon all kinds of contemporary matters which would perhaps have eluded a less practised or perceptive eye. The title-quote for this paper, 'notorious abominations', for example, derives from an article highlighting the defective design of roofs commonly used on cheap speculative housing being erected in the 1840s.[27] Instead of draining rainwater towards gutters at the front and back of a terrace of houses, these 'valley roofs' used every party wall as an apex to a long series of ridge and valley roofs, with gutters running in every valley which ran centrally from front to back of every house. The design was fundamentally flawed, since if for any reason downpipes became blocked – with autumn leaves, for example – inundations would invariably occur in inaccessible locations in the middle of the building, and the preventable result was damp, damage, collapsed ceilings, rot and unhealthy living conditions for those inhabiting the garret floor, and even those inhabiting the floor below. A simple design fault could result in the rapid deterioration of new houses into slums.

On another occasion, Godwin sketched and measured the narrow aperture available for cooking in a typical working-class home.[28] The family occupied the parlour of a house which had originally been designed for a single family, but which in 1863 was in multiple occupation, with a family in every room. Godwin's concern for the experience of women attempting to cook meat and two vegetables for family meals on a small fireplace was not confined to the inconvenience, the smuts, smoke and smell, or even the likelihood of frustration resulting in domestic strife. Godwin also mentioned the additional costs incurred by the poor who took food instead to the local bake-house, the insanitary nature of many of these places, the poor nutritional value of food overcooked in so doing, and the ruination of its flavour. The sketch accompanying the article was made by Godwin himself, light and rather scratchy as was his customary style: not a great work of art, but designed to convey to ignorant contemporaries the realities of ordinary lives. Another of his illustrations featured the water butt he found in the basement of a house in Gray's Inn Lane in 1856, contaminated with sewage from the adjacent cesspool.[29]

Godwin was perhaps one of the earliest social investigators to enter the homes of the poor without social disgust. These sketches were made during a rolling programme of personal slum visits that Godwin reported in the journal, during the 1850s, 1860s and 1870s. Unlike other investigators, as far as we know he used no form of disguise during these journeys. He was sometimes accompanied by John Brown, a working illustrator, who would sketch scenes they witnessed – like a Spitalfields couple weaving by tallow candlelight white watered silk for society wedding dresses, while their seven children slept in beds made up on the bare floorboards; or a bed-sitting room in Whitechapel where an entire family lived and slept while the coffin of a dead child occupied the only table.[30]

There is a hint that Godwin's revelations concerning life in slum tenements caused friction with his employers, and that he was pressured into lowering the volume of his indignation, as a result of displeasure from above.[31] But Godwin continued to report nevertheless: conditions in Sheffield were covered, for example, by way of the publication of his own address to the large audience at the Social Science Congress in Sheffield in 1865:

> He had felt surprise at the death rate in Sheffield, but he had ceased to experience that feeling after a walk in the town. He proceeded to say that he was sorry to make the remark he should make, and he did not wish it to be thought that the Social Science Association had come to Sheffield to find fault; but if such were the case, he hoped that the blame would be put upon his shoulders, and not upon the Society generally. He had been through the courts of Pea-croft, of White-croft, and of Hollis-croft. What he had seen there would of itself more than account for the terrific death rate which they had heard of that day. In one court, in which were seven houses, each having two rooms, there were sixty-two people. The pavements were broken, and the stagnant water and refuse remained about them . . . they were half-starved for water . . . [and] for the whole of those sixty two persons there was but one convenience and that had neither door nor seat! . . . He had spoken warmly because he felt warmly, and he expressed a strong hope that something would be done to remove so crying a disgrace . . . where life and progress were concerned, money should not be allowed to prevent the right work.[32]

The tone here is nearer to Godwin's speaking voice than to his written style, and one gains the impression of a doughty humanitarian. As one contemporary observed: 'Mr Godwin is a gentleman who is not to be deterred from his philanthropic exertions by the stubbornness of aldermen or the ignorance of overseers'.[33]

Godwin's evident anger at the state of things was not politically motivated in a party sense. A 'queen and country' man, he expressly excluded all party political matters from his pages, and would have no one breach the rule. He complained, occasionally in identifiable detail, of 'card castle architects and dirt pie builders', and abhorred the operation of dishonest or exploitative practices of any kind, in an industry in which these were a byword. Perceiving that greed militated against all the journal stood for, Godwin criticized his own times in rhyme:

When party broils and wars of creed are rife,
When rulers shirk the laws of human life,
When duty means the greed for private wealth,
You'll likely find a blighted public health.[34]

Godwin was unafraid of confronting unpleasant truths. On at least one occasion, *The Builder* featured an entire editorial on human excrement, introduced, like the detritus in *Our Mutual Friend*, by means of gold: this time that supposed by country folk to pave London streets. The editorial drew attention to the gold buried beneath the streets in the form of financial investment in:

> the gas-mains which thread the substratum in every direction, like the veins beneath the skin of this Giant of a capital of ours, and the sewers, which are but the bricken intestines packed within the huge bowels of this same Monster of a metropolis . . . we now come to inquire what amount of money must it have taken to fashion the enormous network of sewerage required to carry off the vast feculent flood of sewage daily provided by the four millions of human beings that make up the aggregate population of the capital.[35]

In the event, discussion of the sewerage itself was held over for the following week, and the reader was treated instead to a lengthy consideration of the composition, state, weight and bulk of this so-called 'feculent flood'. The headline for the piece was 'The Cloaca Maxima of the Metropolis Magna'. Let those consider this who think our own era free from taboo subjects.

It is not possible to do justice here to the contents of a forty-year run of *The Builder*, even when one attempts to confine discussion to an apparently discrete topic such as public health. In reality, public health is not at all a discrete subject in *The Builder*: it is pervasive, ubiquitous. Concern for the health of the public arises on almost every page. It is, however, possible to enumerate for you some of the fields in which environment, architecture and public health surface together in *The Builder*. A short chronology of selected issues offers a means of conveying something of the profusion to which allusion has been made. Our indexes will shortly provide a key to the richness of illustration on matters of public health, such as hospitals, schools, cesspools, overcrowding, water supply and sewer design.

In the 1840s we find articles on matters such as public conveniences; parks as urban lungs; overcrowding; intra-mural burial; prisons; working-class housing; bad bricklaying and dangerous structures; domestic drainage and water supplies; the dangers of cesspools; window taxation and the lack of light in poor homes; the provision of public and workplace baths; sewer gas and the introduction of traps in soil pipes and sewers; road surfaces; the prevention of contagion; the health of towns; nutrition; several pleas for centralization urban planning authorities for major towns; insanitary workplaces; public washhouses; industrial diseases; the use of air bricks for ventilation; air pollution; dust; the preservation of open spaces in urban areas; sewer construction – particularly the egg-shaped variety; cholera; the enclosing of open sewers; contamination of water supplies by sewage; model lodging houses; slum clearances; embanking the Thames; street sweeping; and the design of lunatic asylums.

In the following decade, these topics are supplemented by references to the dangers of jerry building in suburban areas; dead dogs in the Thames; insanitary accommodation for farm animals, particularly in urban districts; the potential dangers to human beings of animal diseases; gymnasia and physical fitness; underground dwellings; the keeping of dead bodies in poor homes prior to burial; insanitary slaughterhouses; the pavilion design of hospitals; inspection of nuisances; bed bugs; model housing design in Europe; human guano; overcrowding and insanitary accommodation in barracks; street improvements; ragged schools; arsenic in wallpaper; noxious trades; smallpox; and the high death rate inside workhouses.

Similar concerns continue to emerge in the 1860s and 1870s, with the addition of insanitary housing for the middle and upper classes; insanitary nurseries for small children; Peabody buildings; back-to-back housing in industrial districts; the repulsive habit of spitting; urban cowsheds and their effluvia; the need for play areas for children; the need for a centralized planning authority for London; dangerous road junctions; institutional laundry design; 'deadly beds' in hospitals; destitution; fever dens; lead poisoning; the behaviour of building materials in fire; Turkish baths; pawnshops as brokers of disease; typhus; pigsties and their human inhabitants; public mortuaries; the unsuitability of flat roofs to our climate; deaths from crushing during crowd panic; and the urgent need for adequate emergency exits in public buildings. The design of workhouse infirmaries, disease mapping, and the dangers of private water supplies are supplemented with concern for high infant mortality; the adulteration and contamination of food; designs for schools, almshouses and cottage hospitals; rural slums and their high death rate; noiseless paving in the vicinity of hospitals; public conveniences for women; street watering; the use of human remains cleared from burial grounds as infill in the foundations of new houses; insanitary mortar made from street sweepings; and discussion of germ theory.

Between 1880 and Godwin's retirement in 1883, *The Builder* reported, in addition, upon urban piggeries, insanitary police cells and seaside hotels, the use of foul unventilated cellars as oakum picking areas for workhouse inmates, and the fatal effects of untrapped soil pipes, even in the homes of wealthy people.[36]

One of the things a modern reader most appreciates about the journal is its editor's evident desire to promote social harmony by means of his own energy and skills. Perceiving architectural journalism as a means of assisting public education on important environmental health-related issues, and of thus aiding sanatory improvement, *The Builder* was published week after week for forty years with the optimistic intention of assisting both processes. The editor's good-heartedness permeates the journal, and leaves one impressed with the humanity, as well as the failings unfailingly exposed, of an era which could both produce the man and appreciate his writings.

George Godwin's work as an editor, journalist and campaigning reformer sets him alongside other great nineteenth-century editors, such as Charles Knight of the *Penny Magazine*, *The Lancet*'s Wakley, Jerrold of *Punch*, Dickens at *Household Words*, the *BMJ*'s Ernest Hart, not forgetting W.T. Stead at the *Pall Mall Gazette*. Godwin's writings as a social investigator, published originally in *The Builder* and later in book form – *London Shadows, Town Swamps and Social Bridges, Another Blow for Life* – place him alongside Mayhew and Booth.[37] In addition, the wood engravings he made himself or commissioned from others to accompany his sanitary reform editorials can be said to have nourished the roots of social realism in Victorian art, from Luke Fildes and Gustav Doré to Van Gogh.[38]

The endeavour has been to examine *The Builder*'s considerable influence in public health reform.[39] We have noted that in some other cases – like London's blue plaques and Shakespeare statue – the journal's effects have lasted on into our own time. The Netley Hospital controversy and the subsequent adoption of pavilion hospital design should alert us to the probability that other instances of *The Builder*'s importance in the communication of information may have been overlooked; we only need recall the building labourers milling around in their hundreds near the empty ground on which the Strand law courts now stand to infer the range of *The Builder*'s bush-telegraph.

The architect Alfred Waterhouse, President of the RIBA, announced Godwin's death to the membership in 1888. Alluding to the fact that the journal's editor had been the Institute's longest-surviving member, Waterhouse marked his passing with words of considerable weight: 'Probably, the cause of sanitary science,' he said, '. . . owes more to [George Godwin] than to any other man'.[40] The present writer, from respect to the many other Victorian public health campaigners, would not press so grand a claim. Nevertheless, it is salutary to observe that in 1888 George Godwin, rather than Chadwick, was honoured in such terms by fellow Victorians. A revaluation of the nineteenth-century movement for public health reform is overdue. It is surely time for the revision of a canon which awards fame and laurels to a single individual when the labours were those of many, and many of those unknown.

Acknowledgements

Without Stephen Lock, Roy Porter and Bill Bynum this piece would not have been written. Thanks are due to Brian Hurwitz, Kathleen Tillotson, Betty Bostetter, Robert Thorne, Lindsay Granshaw, Peter Bartrip, Tony King, Anne Summers and descendants of the Godwin family for information, advice, discussion or verification of important points, or for the loan of manuscript material. I also wish to thank staff at the RIBA Library, the British Library, Bloomsbury, the Institute of Historical Research, the Builder Group, the Wellcome Institute and the National Museum of Labour History, Manchester.

Notes

1. S.S. Sprigge, *The Life and Times of Thomas Wakley*, London, 1897. B. Bostetter, Manuscript chapters of a forthcoming biography of Thomas Wakley. In preparation.

2. *Builder* 1888, 75–7.

3. *Builder* 1888, 75–7.

4. A.D. King, 'George Godwin and the Art Union of London, *Victorian Studies* 1964, VIII(2), 101–30.

5. G. Godwin, *Essay on Concrete*, Institute of British Architects Prize Essay, 1836. For the Royal Gold Medal presentation, see *Proceedings* of the Royal Society of British Architects 19.3.1881, 235–55.

6. A letter survives, dated 21 June 1863, in which Dickens addressed Godwin as 'My dear Godwin'. The great Dickens scholar Kathleen Tillotson, editor of several of the novels, and of the Pilgrim edition of his letters, informs me that this was 'almost his most familiar form of address'. The letter provides good evidence that the men knew and liked each other. Personal communication with Prof. Kathleen Tillotson, 13.9.1986. For Godwin's investigative journalism on the lives of the poor see A.D. King, Introduction to G. Godwin, *Town Swamps and Social Bridges* [London, 1859] Leicester/NY, 1972, p.16. See also Godwin's own books: G. Godwin, *London Shadows*, London, 1854; *Town Swamps and Social Bridges* London, 1859; *Another Blow for Life*, London, 1864. The bulk of material published in these volumes had previously appeared in *The Builder*.

7. *Builder* 1848, p.1. See also *Builder* title pages 1848–83.

8. A.D. Brundage, *England's Prussian Minister: Edwin Chadwick and the Politics of Government Growth 1832–54*, Pennsylvania University Park/London, 1989. C. Webster, *The Victorian Public Health Legacy: A Challenge to the Future*, Birmingham, 1990.

9. U. Henriques, *Before the Welfare State: Social Administration in Early Industrial Britain*, London/NY, 1979, 128.

10. The labours of others, notably Henry Austin, ought also to be recognized to a greater degree than is at present the case.

11. A.D. King, Introduction to G. Godwin, *Town Swamps and Social Bridges* [London, 1859] Leicester/NY, 1972, 16.

12. *Builder* 1860, 241; 1872, 250.

13. To give only three eminent examples, see the high incidence of citations of *Builder* material in works of scholars such as H.J. Dyos, Donald Olsen and J. Summerson. The Builder Project's volume, R. Richardson and R. Thorne, *The Builder Illustrations: The Godwin Years, 1843–83*, is currently in preparation and will be published jointly by the Builder Group, English Heritage and the Institute of Historical Research in 1992, with a foreword by HRH Prince Charles.

14. Several of the following, who represent only a small number of those worked on *Builder* illustrations, also exhibited at the Royal Academy: Edmund Evans, Ebenezer Landells, Birket Foster, W.J. Linton, Orlando Jewitt, George Truefitt, George Scharf, George Measom. For further details see Note 13 above. See also Celina Fox, 'Wood

Engravers and The City', in I.B. Nagel and F.S. Schwarzbach, *Victorian Artists and the City*, Oxford, 1980, 4–6.

15. H.A. Cox, *These Stones*, London, 1937, 75.

16. A.D. King, Introduction to G. Godwin, *Town Swamps and Social Bridges* [London 1859] Leicester/NY 1972, 11 citing *The Times* 30.1.1888.

17. Operative Society of Bricklayers Membership Certificate. National Museum of Labour History, Manchester.

18. *Builder* 1875, 35.

19. *Builder* 1845, 601. Other instances of this sort of statement appear in *The Builder* 1870, 709; 1871, 45; 1874, 533; 1875, 871; 1880, 107; 1881, ii, 283.

20. *Builder* 1864, 206–8. See also R. Richardson, 'George Godwin of the Builder', *Visual Resources* (Harvard, USA) 1989, VI, 121–40.

21. Mark Swenarton: *Artisans and Architects: The Ruskinian Tradition in Architectural Thought*, London, 1989, 68–9.

22. A.D. King, 'Hospital Planning: revised thoughts on the Origin of the Pavilion Principle in England', *Medical History* 1966, X(4), 360–73.

23. A.D. King, 'Hospital Planning: revised thoughts on the Origin of the Pavilion Principle in England', *Medical History* 1966, X(4), 366.

24. Correspondence between Florence Nightingale and George Godwin which had survived in the Godwin family has recently been stolen. Personal communication with family members.

25. F. Nightingale, *Notes on Hospitals*, London, 1859.

26. *Builder* 1879, 47; 1879, 228–9.

27. *Builder* 1844, 344.

28. *Builder* 1863, 149.

29. *Builder* 1856, 157.

30. *Builder* 1853, 257; 1853, 225.

31. H.A. Cox, *These Stones*, London, 1937, 75.

32. *Builder* 1864, 724.

33. Review quoted from the journal *Bell's Messenger*, quoted at the back of Godwin's book *Another Blow for Life*, London, 1864.

34. *Builder* 1875, 780.

35. *Builder* 1875, 1073.

36. See the Builder Project volume mentioned in Note 13 above, and *The Builder*'s own annual index pages.

37. See Godwin's publications listed in Note 6 above.

38. One of the engravers of Godwin's slum views was William Luson Thomas who later founded the *Graphic* and commissioned Luke Fildes's famous image of applicants for admission to a Casual Ward, 'Houseless and Hungry', as a wood engraving for the first edition, and which caused a furore when it was exhibited in oils at the Royal Academy in 1874. See also Celina Fox, 'The Development of Social Reportage in English Periodical Illustration', *Past and Present* 1977, 74(19), 90–111; Ronald Pickvance, *English Influences on Vincent Van Gogh*, Catalogue of an Exhibition, Arts Council of Great Britain, 1974/5.

39. Anthony King set the foundation for the modern appreciation of Godwin as a public health reformer. See notes 4, 11 and 22 above, and see A.D. King, 'Another Blow for Life: George Godwin and the Reform of Working Class Housing', *Architectural Review* 1964, 136(814), 448–52.

40. *Proceedings of the Royal Institute of British Architects*, 9.2.1888. The event was reported in *The Builder* 1888, 100.

6

Social diseases? Crime and medicine in the Victorian press

Michael Harris

A long walk from the prison cell to the horse-drawn scaffold (looking, as one reporter at Stafford put it, like a huge piece of agricultural machinery); some raucous shouts from distant parts of a vast and almost silent crowd; a few fluttering breaths under the hood which was drawn over his face; and the story of Dr William Palmer, the Rugeley poisoner, was abruptly terminated. For the newspaper readers of 1856 who had been following the revelations of his life and exploits with exceptional interest, the endless melodrama continued, although with a different cast of characters. Already the copycat poisoning by William Dove at Leeds had begun to absorb the attention of the public at large and, as ever, there was no shortage of less celebrated murders in the hyperactive coverage of the newspaper press.

This paper will circle around the major English poisoning cases involving Drs Palmer and Smethurst which blew with gale force through the mid-Victorian periodicals. Both the period and the subject have received some close scrutiny from scholars in the fields of literature and history who have identified, in the 1850s and 1860s, sometimes with manic specificity, a major shift in the character of English life and culture.[1] One of the latest of these, Thomas Boyle, in his stimulating and sensationally titled study, *Black Swine in the Sewers of Hampstead*, has used a selection of newspaper police reports and examples of sensation fiction to suggest that something was changing in the *Zeitgeist* at mid-century.[2] My aim is rather different and certainly more modest although it relates to this large notion at various points. I hope in the course of these remarks to suggest how medicine was represented within the generalist newspapers published in London and how the coverage of a particular kind of criminal act was part of a dynamic process in which medical issues were a crucial element. Far from being locked into the pages of heavyweight journals, health and medicine achieved a substantial presence in the pages of the weekly and daily press, and the material had a particular force in the construction of the Victorian reader's view of society.

One major difficulty in attempting this sort of analysis arises from the complexity and variety of the printed serials in circulation. In London, and increasingly outside it, there developed a broad spectrum of newspapers and periodicals through which flowed a torrent of miscellaneous, overlapping and often discordant material. Within this dense mass, which has created a high level of bibliographical vertigo, the position of individual titles and the character of their content was directly related to the timing of their publication – in fact, to their periodicity. At one end of the temporal scale stood the slow-motion quarterlies and monthlies whose tone of considered judgement developed in tandem with the involvement of a variety of special, most notably professional, interests. At the other were the pell-mell dailies inextricably caught up in a recurrent programme of deadlines and continuously reconstructing the categories of formula publishing – politics, business and crime among others.

Between these extremes lay the weeklies, facing both ways in publishing terms through a capacity to support both specialist and generalist material. Weekly publication could also provide access to different sectors of the market. *The Lancet* and the *London Medical Gazette* (later the *Medical Times and Gazette*) catered for a primarily professional readership which lay within the sphere of influence of the respectable monthlies. On the other hand, the *Medical Adviser* in the 1820s and the *Doctor* in the 1830s, with their emphasis on self-help diagnosis and treatment, were designed for a mainly working-class audience. The pragmatic interest in medicine at this level is also visible in the content of the most successful of the generalist weeklies, the Sunday papers established in mid-century under the names of Edward Lloyd and G.W.M. Reynolds. Both were beneficiaries of a massive volume of medical advertising[3] and during the 1840s *Lloyd's* engaged in an active dialogue with its readers on issues of personal health. Within this vortex of print, medical science had a significant presence. However, in the generalist papers the material remained largely unfocused and was never consolidated in a separately identified category – unlike, for example, reports on the railways or sport. Medical issues continued to crop up in other settings and consequently became a pervasive but unstable element in the newspapers' carefully structured commentary on events.

Nowhere was the cross-over between forms of information and comment more evident in mid-century than in the relationship between medicine and crime. The amount of space devoted to the coverage of crime, particularly as it was dealt with in the courts, was enormous. Whatever the variation in detail the papers, popular or respectable, daily or weekly, sorted out and identified their routine coverage in much the same way. In each case the London police courts formed a separate and often substantial part of the allotted space. The material, subdivided by location, was often divided again with subheadings identifying the nature of the case. From the *Daily Telegraph* of Wednesday 5 January 1859: 'Mansion House. Benevolence', 'Bow Street. Garroting', 'Marlborough Street. Assault on a Girl', 'Marylebone. Extraordinary Charge – Throwing an Infant out of Window Under the Alleged Influence of a Dream', 'Westminster. Desperate Outrages', and so on. Although the queue of individuals passing through the columns of the newspaper included some particularly newsworthy characters (an Ethiopian serenader on a manslaughter charge or a Russian princess down on her luck)[4] the spectacle, as Boyle remarks, is, in the end, a depressing one. To the police reports have to be added the regular newspaper coverage of the Central Criminal Court, the Civil Courts and the Assize Circuits as well as the reports of inquests held at miscellaneous public houses. Court hearings of any kind outside London were also grist to the mills of the weeklies and dailies, and in this way a large volume of space was filled in each issue of each title. Even so, as in the great set-piece cases of the poisoners, the material could burst its boundaries and become the dominant feature of papers individually and collectively. The Palmer trial at the Old Bailey in May 1856 lies across the content of the Victorian press like the stratum of burnt material from the Fire of London which provides a temporal marker for archaeologists in the City.

The presence of this material can only partly be explained by the immediate pressures of reader demand. It also had, like the coverage of parliament that choked the pages of the Victorian papers in the course of every session, a semi-formal status as a public record. Publicity through the press was held to be as crucial to the operation of the legal system as the notional application of public opinion was to the political. This sometimes appeared in the treatment of journalists. At Palmer's execution the representatives of the provincial and metropolitan papers were to have been provided with a specially constructed stand close enough to the scaffold to catch his final words, until the order was rescinded locally.[5] Criticism of the newspaper coverage came from all directions, not least from the courts themselves. But although the way in which the court reports were collected and edited remains largely below the surface, the material, constantly winnowed by public scrutiny, seems to have been reasonably accurate. Letters were published correcting matters of fact while the papers themselves were sometimes involved in obscure editorial interventions. An inquest report published in *Lloyd's* was corrected in a letter to *The Times*, the facts were checked with the coroner by a member of *Lloyd's* staff and the fault acknowledged in the paper a few days later.[6] This routine sharing out of information gave the papers a collective importance in relation to the law and they could, in some respects, be represented as a legitimate component in the administration of justice.

The presentation of material generated by the courts was not always a straightforward process. In one area in particular the tensions inherent in the relations of official and commercial organizations could create difficulty. This concerned the publication of hard-core medical evidence. In the routine coverage, the newspapers were willing to lay before the public the most horrifying circumstances of the cases they reported, though with some occasional flinching. Thomas Boyle has suggested that the weight and character of this material, containing a view of Victorian society in which dreadful cruelty and terrible abuses of personal authority were uppermost, amounted to the construction of a subversive counterculture.[7] This seems to me to contain a misunderstanding of the newspaper as well as of the function of the reports. In the concentrated form of a collection of cuttings, which formed Boyle's primary source, the coverage inevitably appeared more threatening than it would have done in the setting of individual issues of the generalist papers. It is certainly useful for the historian to read about the Whitechapel murders in conjunction with reports of the Australian cricket tour, and the response of contemporary readers who, after all, were involved in the construction of their own sense of reality by a process of selection and exclusion, must have been substantially modified. It was equally possible to gloss over crime as over the other carefully identified categories of politics, business or sport. Perhaps as importantly, the often dreadful detail was presented through the normative context of the court hearing. As part of the semi-official record, the material became as much a prop to the existing system of authority as a mechanism of subversion.

Editorial decisions about the publication of detailed medical evidence related to this issue, and its inclusion or exclusion, involved several interrelated considerations. The problem was partly one of technical detail which was often beyond the grasp of judges and juries as well as shorthand writers and newspaper readers.[8] However, editorial decisions were complicated by the need to work along the confusing boundary between morbid curiosity and public outrage. In a general setting, medical material could cause some uneasiness. During the 1830s each issue of *The Doctor* was headed up by a half-page engraving, usually showing some awful medical condition. This was too much for some readers who complained that the illustrations were 'too exclusively professional, and calculated rather to excite disgust than give practical instruction'.[9] In his notice to subscribers the editor agreed to exclude such material but as subsequent issues carried representations of 'Amputation at the Hip Joint' and 'Forcible Separation of the Entire Arm from the Body' it is hard to see how he kept to this undertaking. In the court reports it seems that when medical evidence was a vital part of a major case neither technicality nor revulsion deterred publication. All the London papers seem to have carried the post-mortem report of Drs Taylor and Rees on the remains of Palmer's alleged victim, John Parsons Cook, and the contents of what Henry Mayhew described as 'jars 1, 2 and 3 of unhappy celebrity'[10] were laid before the public in full. In this instance publication was integral to the coverage of the inquest.

At other times publication of medical detail was highly equivocal and seldom more so than in the case of two wealthy young transvestites accused in 1870 of unnatural practices.[11] Known as the case of 'The Men in Petticoats', medical evidence of homosexuality was central to the prosecution. Full details of the police surgeon's initial examination were published in *Reynolds's* under the heading 'The Men in Petticoats – Horrible and Revolting Disclosures'.[12] In spite of heavy criticism from other publications, including the *Saturday Review* and 'that half-penny hypocrite' the *Echo*, *Reynolds's* provided an equally full restatement of the rectal examination in reporting the trial the following year.[13] The paper's defence of its actions was, as might be expected, equivocal. It was based mainly on its duty to give readers as full and explicit an account of events as possible, suggesting that 'publication of such details as those to which we now especially allude, could not do any harm to those who are aware that such crimes exist, and could not be understood by those who are ignorant on the subject'.[14] An indication of the way in which medical evidence as published in the newspapers straddled the worlds of science and sensationalism, even of pornography, was provided in the form of a pub entertainment in which men dressed as women pretended to be giving graphic sexual testimony in court.[15]

The editorial selection of cases for inclusion in the newspaper reports brought into view a sequence of doctors, surgeons, chemists and quacks. Often facing charges of manslaughter by prescription or treatment, or defending malpractice libels, the respectability of this erratic sub-group gave it some prominence. For the most part, the doctors in court were not involved in circumstances which were extreme or dramatic enough to attract further newspaper interest. However, in the cases of Drs Palmer and Smethurst, the supposed involvement of members of a respectable and skilled profession in the most ominous form of murder made them, during the course of a few months, into national, even international, figures. This did not provoke any general critique of the medical profession although it gave some point to the continuing demand for a more careful check on the qualifications for admission and for the weeding out of individuals such as those who, according to *Lloyd's*, squeezed in 'by some little back-door Scotch university'.[16] The slightly queasy optimism later expressed by Arthur Griffiths that 'the doctors might decimate the human race, if their morality did not stand so high'[17] was shared by the newspapers of the 1850s. The poisoners themselves were presented as individuals with fatally flawed characters rather than as maverick doctors – Palmer as gambler and manipulator of life insurance and Smethurst as a bigamist. Smethurst's interest in hydrotherapy and his spell as editor of the *Water-Cure Journal* were never identified.

On the other side of the court the poison cases brought into sharp focus the doctors appearing at each stage of the legal process as expert witnesses. Their collective position in this setting was always difficult and the newspapers reflected the problem with some clarity. During the trials, specialists employed by the defence were lined up against those for the prosecution, presenting what appeared to be flatly contradictory evidence in barely comprehensible terms. The court became the area for what the *Daily Telegraph* described as 'the clashing *dicta* of the scientific professions'[18] and the system was criticized in the newspapers as well as by the doctors themselves, only too well aware of the bad public image presented through the press. A defensive statement in the *Medical Times* during the Palmer case admitted that 'there is no home we enter, where this wretched business is discussed, in which we do not hear the observation: What shocking discrepancies among the Medical witnesses! What a poor exhibition the doctors have made of themselves!'[19] The same weekly was particularly annoyed by the process of cross-examination: 'the unavoidable intricacies of the subject afford means for half educated and pert attorneys, or for conceited and shallow barristers, to browbeat and perplex the Medical witness'.[20] In court, medicine was subordinated to the law and the image of the confused specialist recurred in the press.

Newspaper coverage of the major poison cases was comprehensive. From the inquests, through the trials, to the implementation or setting aside of the sentences, a full record of the proceedings was linked to editorial comment, special reports and a substantial amount of correspondence. The poison cases, like the medical evidence itself, lay across the boundaries of the sensational and the scientific and this could cause difficulties for the specialist medical papers, particularly those caught up in the dynamics of weekly publication. The *Medical Times* displayed the effects of the cross-currents in its ambivalent approach to the Palmer case. Anxious not to lose out on its early notoriety, editorials hinted at special access to information deliberately withheld.[21] As the case developed momentum the *Medical Times* began to express a particular and legitimate interest in its implications for medical jurisprudence. The paper announced its intention of 'coolly and dispassionately examining, by the light of science, the evidence of murder as revealed by physiological, pathological or chemical investigation'.[22] In the event the paper hired a special reporter and devoted an unprecedented fifty-six columns to the hearing at the Old Bailey.

As the newspapers sifted the evidence and put together a composite picture of the cases, they themselves became actors in the events they described. This was not just an interplay of style and content, between what has been described as technique and message. The interaction was more pragmatic and visible. Thirty publications were said to be represented at the Rugeley inquests and according to the *Daily Telegraph* the streets of the town were full of artists, many presumably employed by the illustrated press.[23] In this setting, contact, not to say conflict, with the principals was almost inevitable. Dr Palmer's brother initiated a libel action against the *Illustrated London News* for an extraordinary attack on his family by the paper's special correspondent, and the move of the trial from Stafford to London was said to be a direct result of the build-up in popular interest through the press.[24] On the other hand, both the Palmer and Smethurst cases hinged on technical medical evidence and the expert witnesses themselves became primary targets in the journalist's search for hot news and background information.

This newsworthiness applied with particular force to Dr Alfred Swaine Taylor, a high-status expert regularly employed by the Treasury on poisoning cases. Taylor was the first Professor of Medical Jurisprudence at Guy's Hospital and author of a standard and often reprinted work on poisons. Like other leading pioneers in toxicology, such as Sir Robert Christison, his appearance in court signalled the seriousness and importance of the case. Unfortunately, in spite of his journalistic experience as editor of the *London Medical Gazette*, Taylor had an image problem and the interplay between medical witness, the court and the press was highlighted in his apparently dismal performances. To some extent Taylor was a victim of circumstances. During the inquest on Palmer's alleged victim, Cook, the coroner took vigorous exception to the fact that the autopsy report from Taylor and Rees appeared in *The Times* before it had been given in evidence.[25] Taylor had released the material to a journalist from the *Morning Post* as the journalist and his colleagues were dashing back to London by train, on the understanding that it would be held back until legitimately released in court. This off-the-record agreement seems to have been adhered to and, in fact, the report was leaked by the police to a local stringer working for *The Times*. Even so, it was an unpromising start to his involvement.

At Palmer's trial in May, undermining Taylor's credibility was crucial to the defence and during cross-examination a good deal was made of an interview he had given to the *Illustrated Times* in January. At that time Taylor had already written to *The Lancet* complaining about some remarks on his evidence at the Cook inquest, and it may have been his wish to put himself in a better light that encouraged him to agree to an interview at his house in London by the dynamic social reporter Henry Mayhew.[26] Mayhew, who was engaged on a series of articles on 'The Number of Suspicious Deaths Occurring in Connection with Life Insurance', had a letter of recommendation from Professor Faraday and carried out his questioning with characteristic thoroughness and good humour. At the trial, some three months after publication, Taylor claimed that the interview had been obtained surreptitiously, that he had not agreed to publication and that his picture which accompanied the text was also unauthorized. He claimed that the paper had caricatured his views (he particularly denied saying 'I would give them enough strychnia before I had done with them') and that the article was 'perfectly disgraceful'. Mayhew's reaction to the publication of the evidence was instantaneous. He wrote a brisk and highly indignant rebuttal of Taylor's claims, point by point, which was immediately published in several London newspapers including *The Times* and the *Daily Telegraph*.[27] With the trial still under way, the *Telegraph* reprinted the original interview verbatim.[28] Taylor seems, as Mayhew himself suggested, to have become 'so confused by his long and rigid cross-examination that he was not exactly aware of the serious charge conveyed in his words'.

Taylor's image in the newspapers was constructed out of a number of elements. To some extent it represented a straight reflection of the proceedings in court where his evidence was made to look decidedly shaky. In the Palmer case he attempted to suggest that his failure to find strychnine in the post-mortem examination of Cook had resulted partly from a process of absorption. This was a highly contentious view that provided a handle for a serious and prolonged attack in the press on his professional competence. In the Smethurst case Taylor went one stage better and claimed to have identified arsenic, which later proved to have been produced by a chemical reaction in his own apparatus. As a leader in the *Daily Telegraph* scathingly remarked, 'the Doctor seems to have brought his arsenic along with him when he came to seek for it; and he was compelled to acknowledge his most grievous error and blunder when his much vaunted copper gauge boiled way in potassium'.[29] Taylor was extremely exposed and he compounded his own difficulties by comments which, at least as reported, were palpably ridiculous. After the interchange in court over the Mayhew interview, he was said to have claimed that 'As regards the effects of strychnia on the human frame, I have no knowledge of my own at all, but I have written a book on the subject'.

The manufacture of Taylor's image in the newspapers was not achieved by a simple reworking of the court proceedings. It was also shaped by the networks of confrontation and alliance outside the court. Within the press the uniformity of coverage of the poison cases was only skin-deep. The respectable editorial position of such papers as *The Times* and the *Illustrated London News* made them more likely to defer to the case for the Crown than either *The Daily Telegraph* or the popular Sundays. *Lloyd's* and *Reynolds's* were habitually opposed to the political establishment and this attitude spilled over to the medical equivalent. One symptom of this was provided by a willingness, shared with the popular specialist weeklies, to give space and credibility to phrenology. Although most of the papers referred to the cast of Palmer's head taken by 'Mr. Bridges, professor of phrenology' immediately after the execution, only *Reynolds's* provided a detailed account of his findings – 'the extreme predominance of secretiveness; his utter want of conscientiousness, and his defect in the higher reflective powers' and so on.[30] Equally, the divisions of status and opinion within the medical profession also came into play. Drs Taylor and Brodie were invariably on the Treasury payroll representing the prosecution, while for personal, professional and ideological reasons Drs Herepath and Lethaby were equally likely to line up for the defence. These positions were not fixed nor mutually exclusive. Lethaby and other doctors supporting the defence in the Palmer and Smethurst cases wrote voluminously to *The Times* in spite of its editorial scepticism. But even so, the lines were drawn and formed part of the hidden agenda within which the representation of the poison cases and of Dr Taylor were put together.

Newspaper coverage of these cases was never confined to the static representation of events. During, and most strikingly after, the sentencing of Palmer and Smethurst the newspapers became engaged in what amounted to the public retrial of both. The ambiguities of the medical evidence as well as the refusal of either to admit guilt allowed the dynamic of the newspaper to come into effect. This was partly a matter of editorial denunciations of Taylor and the expression of doubts about the uses of forensic science. However, it also involved the orchestration of a large amount of correspondence. As well as the major figures in the field of toxicology, whether appearing as medical witnesses or not, large numbers of doctors, patients and lay observers wrote to the papers on the primary issue of tests for poisons and the identification of symptoms. Case histories poured in and the confrontation of medical witnesses in court was duplicated in the press, greatly to the advantage of the defence. The potential interaction of newspaper and court could also operate in this area. During Palmer's trial a letter to the *Daily Telegraph*, signed simply 'Medicus', provided the details of a case in which a patient suffering from tetanic spasms displayed the symptoms of strychnine poisoning. The following day a letter from Palmer's solicitor, Smith, was published, urgently requesting 'Medicus' to contact him at the court. 'Truth, justice, sense and human life require the fullest investigation,' he wrote. It is not clear whether there was any response.[31]

Just before the implementation of the death sentence Smith, in an open letter to the newspapers, rehearsed the ambiguities of the medical evidence and pleaded for a stay of execution, at least until the scientific controversy had been resolved.[32] He clearly felt that Palmer's last and best hope was the press. Although, as *The Times* suggested, Palmer made a dubious hero, he began to accumulate some public sympathy.[33] The silent crowd at his execution was at least a symbol of the doubts and fears awoken by the newspapers about forensic science as an instrument of justice. In Smethurst's case, the charge led by the *Daily Telegraph* certainly contributed to his sudden pardon, a move which the paper claimed represented a virtual capitulation of the legal system to the popular press.[34]

The comprehensive newspaper coverage of the set-piece poisoning cases carried with it a view of medicine and medical science which was far from clear-cut. The peculiar sort of role reversal by which, in some papers, the accused became the hero and the expert medical witness the villain makes the image flicker and lose definition. However, the trials of Palmer and Smethurst were far from isolated phenomena. Secret poisoning had been high on the agenda of the generalist newspapers since the 1840s and over time the elements of poison and forensic medicine came into equilibrium. To some extent, the framework for the extended coverage was provided by the economic circumstances of the press itself. This appears most fully in the overblown treatment of the Palmer case which dominated the papers in the year following the repeal of the stamp tax. The removal of this heavy burden led to the immediate construction of a stratum of cheap publications, of which the *Daily Telegraph* was a prime example. With cover prices falling across the press, competition became progressively fiercer and an increasingly urgent search for readers began. It was at this moment that Dr Palmer emerged from the shadows and the hyperactive response of the newspapers can be linked to financial self-interest as well as social concern. Although it is impossible to sort out the details of cause and effect, some newspapers were doing very well during the first half of 1856 when the Palmer case was on the boil. When the *Illustrated Times* published a 'Rugeley Number' its circulation was said to have doubled to 400,000 copies.[35] *Lloyd's* announced that, as a result of increased demand, an order had been placed for two of the enormous, six-feeder Hoe presses, while the *Daily Telegraph* claimed that its 'enormous circulation' prevented any alteration to its publication schedules.[36] The knock-on effect of the newspapers' commercial interest in poisoning was ironically identified in *Punch*. 'The "Poisoning Cases",' it suggested, 'have been, of course, a delicious hope for the paragraph-mongers, who have been literally living upon poison for nearly a month, and who get a fresh dinner by every fresh discovery of a little arsenic.'[37]

The build-up in the coverage of poisoning was not simply a commercial device. The newspapers needed to sustain their interactive relationship with their readers and in the treatment of poison they found a means of identifying and redirecting a series of larger fears and preoccupations. The unsubstantiated increase in secret poisoning not only appeared to threaten the security of the individual in the privacy of his or her own home but to endanger the entire fabric of society. Like garroting in the 1860s, poisoning became the focus for what has been called media panic.[38] This was orchestrated in various ways through the press. The regular accumulation of such special headings as 'More Poisonings – Wilful Murder at Deptford' or 'Horrible Tragedy – Another Case of Wholesale Poisoning' was not limited to the popular Sundays and was combined with a consistently gloomy social prognosis. This is a 'Poisoning Aera' announced the *Pictorial Times* in 1847, receiving unexpected support for this view from Dr Taylor in the preface to his book on poisons.[40] The commentary which ran alongside this coverage, particularly during the major trials, was usually expressed in the most lurid terms. Thomas Boyle has demonstrated the intricate cross-referencing between crime reporting and sensation fiction, particularly after 1855, and it is sometimes hard to separate the elements in the heightened language of the press. 'The poison fiend is abroad,' wrote a contributor to the *London Journal* in 1856, 'the fell spirit of the Borgias is stalking through English society'.[41] Even the *Medical Times* felt inclined to refer to the 'dreadful epidemic of wickedness which now overspreads the land like a pestilence'.[42]

Such highly coloured representations were interspersed with a broader analysis in which secret poisoning was linked to a variety of social problems. In the context of fears about the breakdown of social organization, the increase of poisoning was often represented in the newspapers as a by-product of the spread of education and information. Once contained within the upper classes, the characteristic practitioners of the art of poisoning had been the Marchioness de Brinvilliers or, more recently, Thomas Wainewright, 'art critic and poisoner'. Now the crime had moved down the social scale and the poisoner had become a more ominous and generalized figure. Poisoning, accidental or deliberate, already underlay the long-running attempts to control the availability of dangerous substances and to prevent the adulteration of food, drink and drugs. In this area the cross-over between the general issues and the specific poisoning cases was particularly clear. The parliamentary committee on adulteration sat during the build-up to Palmer's trial, and Dr Taylor, as expert witness, provided a personal link between the two. A direct association was made in the *Daily Telegraph* in commenting on the ludicrous notion of 'a whole county frightened from its property at the bare contemplation of the Rugeley poisoning case, and at the same time victimised in detail by the slow process [of poisoning] patronised by a band of knavish grocers in the locality'.[43]

Poison seeped through the newspapers of the mid-nineteenth century and poisoning assumed a presence that cannot be explained in terms of a statistical increase in this form of crime. Presented in the newspapers through commentaries that abounded in the metaphors of disease, poisoning stood out from other crimes, partly because of the degree of premeditation required, but primarily because of its subtlety. Both the materials used and the mind capable of applying them seemed to set the poisoner apart from other criminals. The mysterious and elusive workings of poison were a familiar subject in the press and they were rehearsed for readers of the *Daily Telegraph* on the first day of Palmer's trial. 'What can be more wonderful than that a drop of clear fluid like prussic acid, a compound of carbon, nitrogen, and hydrogen, ingredients existing simple in the first instance . . . should still all that subtle machinery of life in a moment. One convulsive shudder, and the brain, was it that of Newton, will cease to think, the senses to feel, the heart to beat, and the limbs to move!'[44]

At the heart of the mystery of poison lay the special difficulty of detection. This was not simply a technical matter. The slow and intimate process involving doctor and patient, husband and wife, and worked out behind closed doors, seemed to open up vistas of unsolved crime and sent a frisson through the press. A leader in *The Times* engaged in some characteristic speculation during the Smethurst case.

> Who can hope to penetrate into the mysteries of this great town? Who can tell what is passing in any one of the dull uniform rows of houses of which London is made up? The true history of a single street would be a more romantic chronicle than any which the novelist has conjured up.[45]

It was detection as the only effective means of deterrence and prevention that brought forensic medicine into play as a bulwark against the 'terrible dexterity' of the poisoner. In their representations of the dreadful threat to the individual and to society, the newspapers were always prepared to throw in the useful reassurance of the progress of medical science. This view of the conflicting forces of crime and chemical analysis sometimes took on a pragmatic, informational form. Material describing tests for poison, sometimes extracted from the mainstream medical journals, appeared in the press as an almost routine adjunct to the major trials. In 1847, during the trial of a Greenwich poisoner, the *Pictorial Times* offered its readers a long illustrated article on the tests for arsenic, claiming that 'the most subtle and intense of criminal agencies is discovered and disarmed by the light of chemistry'.[46] During the lead-in to Palmer's trial the *Daily Telegraph* attempted 'to prepare the public mind' for the special medical evidence by publication of some equally reassuring material on chemical and other tests.[47]

This capacity of forensic medicine to reveal the hidden secrets of murder was also celebrated in the newspapers in more heightened language and with almost mystical fervour. As the medical scientist moved into the area previously reserved for the action of divine providence, some of the attributes of revelation were also transferred. In an article entitled 'Science in the Witness Box', published in the *Examiner* in 1856 and reprinted in *The Times*, full expression was given to this notion.[48]

According to the writer, time could no longer release the poisoner 'from the horror of the day that may come, when in the face of his fellow-men the very dead shall be drawn up out of the grave to bear witness against him'. The 'natural language' of science had acquired the power of interpretation and 'in a clear voice the murdered wife has spoken', while 'blood now literally cries out of the dust'. Such language was directly in line with that of Henry Fielding in his tract *Examples of the Interposition of Providence in the Detection and Punishment of Murder* (1750). A hundred years later forensic medicine was overtaking divine intervention. As one journalist claimed, medical knowledge was reducing killing by poison 'to the level of a vulgar murder perpetrated by the knife, the bludgeon, or the pistol of the common assassin'.[49] Such uninformed optimism may have borne down on the expert witnesses displaying various kinds of human fallibility in court, and public disappointment certainly sharpened up the criticism of Dr Taylor.

The interactions of crime, medicine and the newspaper in mid-Victorian England were complex and layered. Running through all sections of the press and moving across the components of individual publications, notions of health and medicine formed part of the continuous interchange between producers and readers. Their presence was focused, in the generalist press, in the coverage of poisoning which, in turn, began to inform the language of the newspapers and to become an integral part of their engagement with contemporary society. The overlapping elements of poisoning, the legal system, news and health were sometimes brought into striking conjunction. In the *Daily Telegraph* a description of the setting for the

Smethurst trial at the Old Bailey was presented with almost allegorical force:

> In that hot, dark, unwholesome arena, within narrow walls, with a sombre roof, and immoveable windows, judge, jury, bar, public, prisoner, and witnesses are jammed together; the windows are twice broken to relieve the half-stifled bench; the witnesses are mounted in a pillory; counsel and attorneys are cribbed in a feverish area; the entire area is a black hole, of which the moral atmosphere is no better than the physical . . . In the midst of fainting, confusion, wrangling, recrimination, bluster, casuistry, jealousy and empiricism was this wretched trail dragged to an end.[50]

The specialist medical periodicals, such as the *British Medical Journal*, geared to the interests and practices of the profession, marked out the frontiers of medical science and provided a locus for profound technical discussion. Their content was, by and large, not intended for, nor easily accessible to the lay reader. Nonetheless, a sense of the shifts in knowledge and approach did find its way into the catch-all content of the generalist newspapers. This essay has attempted to indicate how the almost universal preoccupation with the details of crime provided one line of public access to notions about the theory and practice of medicine.

Notes

1. Richard Altick provides a useful account of the Palmer and Smethurst cases in *Victorian Studies in Scarlet*, London: J.M. Dent, 1972. However, in his most recent work, *Evil Encounters; Two Victorian Sensations*, London: John Murray, 1987, he tries to demonstrate that the massive coverage of two minor cases in 1861 marked a specific point of cultural change.

2. Thomas Boyle, *Black Swine in the Sewers of Hampstead*, London: Hodder and Stoughton, 1990, p.37. Boyle's cultural analysis is of considerable interest and any reservations expressed below have been more than offset by the benefits I have received from his work.

3. The most effective discussion of medical advertising in the popular Sundays appears in Virginia Berridge, 'Popular Journalism and Working Class Attitudes, 1854–1886', unpublished Ph.D. thesis, 3 vols, University of London, 1976.

4. *The Times*, Monday 8 June 1857; *Reynolds's Newspaper*, Sunday 10 February 1856.

5. *Reynolds's Newspaper*, Sunday 15 June 1856; *Daily Telegraph*, Monday 16 June 1856.

6. *Lloyd's Weekly Newspaper*, Sunday 11 April 1847.

7. Boyle, op. cit., pp.25, 63. The large collection of cuttings on which his work is based was compiled by a retired surgeon whose interest was probably more clinical than political; motivated more, perhaps, by a form of scientific curiosity than by fear.

8. For some conventional comments on the inability of juries to cope with detailed technical evidence see *Daily Telegraph*, Saturday 20 August 1859; Tuesday 23 August 1859.

9. *Doctor*, Wednesday 27 March 1833.

10. *Daily Telegraph*, Thursday 22 May 1856.

11. The civil case against Boulton and Park was initiated in the Court of Queen's Bench in 1870. The hearing was completed in 1871 when both were acquitted.

12. *Reynolds's Newspaper*, Sunday 24 August 1870.

13. ibid., Sunday 14 May 1871; Sunday 21 May 1871.

14. ibid., Sunday 5 September 1870.

15. Boyle, op. cit. p. 209.

16. *Lloyd's Weekly Newspaper*, Sunday 6 January 1856.

17. Arthur Griffiths, *Mysteries of Police and Crime*, London, 3 vols, n.d., vol. 3, p.58.

18. *Daily Telegraph*, Thursday 15 May 1856.

19. *Medical Times*, Saturday 28 June 1856.

20. ibid., Saturday 22 March 1856. For a valuable study of a related area see Roger Smith, *Trial by Medicine; Insanity and Responsibility in Victorian Trials*, Edinburgh: Edinburgh University Press, 1981.

21. *Medical Times*, Saturday 12 January 1856; Saturday 26 January 1856.

22. ibid., Saturday 22 March 1856.

23. Boyle, op. cit. p.73; *Daily Telegraph*, Saturday 19 January 1856.

24. The attack, which received some attention in other sections of the press, appeared in the *Illustrated London News*, Saturday 19 January 1856. Notice of the libel action and some editorial distancing from the original comments in Saturday 2 February 1856.

25. What follows is based on the reports of the inquest proceedings with some additional commentary in *The Times* and *Daily Telegraph*, Monday 14 January 1856.

26. Mayhew's activities after 1852, when he completed his extraordinary study of the London labour market, are very obscure, E.P. Thompson and Eileen Yeo, *The Unknown Mayhew*, London: Merlin Press, 1971, p.48. It seems that part at least of his considerable energies was deployed through the press and that his association with the *Illustrated Times*, possibly owned by his brother Augustus, fills in part of the picture. His interview with Taylor appeared on Saturday 26 January 1856. Taylor's evidence at the Palmer trial appeared in many papers including *Daily Telegraph*, Tuesday 20 May 1856.

27. *The Times* and *Daily Telegraph*, Wednesday 21 May 1856.

28. *Daily Telegraph*, Thursday 3 May 1856.
29. ibid., Saturday 20 August 1858.
30. *Reynolds's Newspaper*, Sunday 22 June 1856.
31. *Daily Telegraph*, Wednesday 21 May 1856.
32. ibid., Tuesday 3 June 1856; *The Times*, Friday 6 June 1856.
33. *The Times*, Thursday 5 June 1856.
34. *Daily Telegraph*, Monday 29 August 1859.
35. Altick, *Victorian Studies*, p.153.
36. *Lloyd's Weekly Newspaper*, Sunday 8 June 1856; *Daily Telegraph*, Wednesday 21 May 1856.
37. *Punch*, Saturday 26 January 1856.
38. A useful account of this phenomenon appears in Rob Sindall, *Street Violence in the Nineteenth Century: Media Panic or Real Danger?*, Leicester, London and New York: Leicester University Press, 1990.
39. *Lloyd's Weekly Newspaper*, Sunday 5 September 1847; Sunday 12 September 1847.
40. Alfred S. Taylor, *On Poisons in Relation to Medical Jurisprudence and Medicine*, London, 1848, p.v; *Pictorial Times*, Saturday 4 December 1847.
41. *London Journal*, Saturday 5 April 1856.
42. *Medical Times*, Saturday 22 March 1856.
43. *Daily Telegraph*, Wednesday 9 April 1856.
44. ibid., Wednesday 14 March 1856.
45. *The Times*, Monday 22 August 1859.
46. *Pictorial Times*, Saturday 14 February 1846.
47. *Daily Telegraph*, Wednesday 14 May 1856.
48. *The Times*, Saturday 26 January 1856.
49. *Daily Telegraph*, Saturday 22 March 1856 (quotation from the *Medical Times*).
50. ibid., Tuesday 23 August 1859.

7

The *British Medical Journal*: a retrospect

Peter Bartrip

A pedant might question whether 1990 really did mark the *British Medical Journal*'s 150th anniversary. After all, the title dates only from 1857. The medical weekly which then adopted the new name had previously gone under three others: the *Provincial Medical and Surgical Journal*, the *Provincial Medical Journal and Retrospect of Medical Sciences* (twice), and the *Association Medical Journal*. What these have in common with the *BMJ* is that they were all, in the time-honoured phrase, 'the organ of the Association', that is, of the British Medical Association or, as it was known between 1832 and 1856, the Provincial Medical and Surgical Association. However, notwithstanding the similarities between their names, this was not true of the *Provincial Medical and Surgical Journal* when its first number appeared over 150 years ago. Although one of its original co-editors, the Worcester physician, Robert Streeten, was a member of the Association's Council, the new journal was an independent commercial speculation, the success of which was totally dependent on sales and advertising revenue. It was published and printed, far from the Association's Worcester power base, in London, where the 'responsible Editor' was its paediatrician founder, the shadowy Irishman, Peter Hennis Green. Streeten was decidedly the second in command. He had little to do with management; as his *Journal* obituary, rather disparagingly put it, he 'only wrote the leading articles'.[1]

Green, who was not even a member of the PMSA when it held its annual meeting in 1840 (though he had joined by the end of the year), was born in Cork, the son of a farmer, in 1803 or 1804. In 1820 he entered Trinity College Dublin as a 'pensioner' (a status which indicated 'moderate' parental income), graduating BA in 1825 and MB in 1829.[2] If Green was the *Journal's* founding father and the presiding genius of its early years, there is little hint of why he was interested in establishing his own medical weekly. Certainly he already had experience of medical journalism for, like several of those who subsequently edited the *BMJ*, he learned his trade on *The Lancet*. At any rate such would seem to be the case, for it is probable that Green was 'Erinensis' who, between 1824 and 1836, was *The Lancet*'s 'man in Dublin'. As such, he was 'the author of a brilliant series of sketches and letters . . . on the Irish medical scene'. Indeed, James Fernandez Clarke, a medical journalist who worked on the early *Lancet*, doubted 'whether any articles which appeared . . . during my connexion with it, had more literary merit than those of 'Erinensis' .' In his autobiography Clarke went so far as to suggest that the Erinensis letters were chiefly responsible for *The Lancet*'s 'power' during the 1820s and 1830s.[3]

The identity of Erinensis was a closely guarded secret to which Clarke could offer no clue. In fact, the first indication that Green and Erinensis were one and the same person was provided by Sir Charles Cameron in his *History of the Royal College of Surgeons in Ireland*. In a brief footnote Cameron states that 'through the courtesy of Dr. [James] Wakley, proprietor of *The Lancet*, I have ascertained that the writer of these letters [Erinensis] was an Irishman, Dr. Herris [*sic*] Green, for eighteen years a member of the staff of *The Lancet*'.[4] If it is assumed that 'Herris' was simply a typographical error, the main question raised by Cameron's note concerns the period of Green's association with *The Lancet*. If this really lasted for eighteen years Green must have been on its staff almost up to the time that he launched the *PMSJ*. There are few details of what he did between 1836 and 1840, though he clearly spent a year or so in Paris pursuing his interest in childhood diseases, a subject on which he published several papers (under his own name) in *The Lancet* during 1837–9. By 1838 he was back in London where he was a witness when Wakley tested John Elliotson's claims for mesmerism. A year later, in a letter to *The Lancet*, Green described himself as that journal's 'sub-editor'. But his long working relationship with Wakley lasted little longer, his final contribution to *The Lancet* appearing in May 1840. At the time of the *PMSJ*'s launch, in the following October, he was lecturer in the diseases of childhood at the

Hunterian School of Medicine in Great Windmill Street, Haymarket.[5]

From the outset Green hoped to forge a link between his journal and the PMSA – hence his choice of title.[6] The Association had some 1200 members in 1840; if a large proportion of these could be induced to subscribe to the *PMSJ* its prospects would be bright. To be sure, the PMSA, which had been founded by Charles Hastings in Worcester in 1832, already had its own publication, the annual *Transactions of the Provincial Medical and Surgical Association.* First published in 1833, it carried scientific, topographical and clinical papers as well as reports of Association business, notably the proceedings of annual meetings. Produced at considerable expense and to a high standard, it was the Association's 'flagship', but in 1840 the PMSA's Council was receptive to the idea of supplementing it with a weekly journal, its only reservation being 'the expense incident to such an undertaking'.[7]

The Lancet's success amply demonstrated that there was a demand for medical weeklies. Although several of those launched in the 1820s and 1830s survived only briefly, the *London Medical Gazette*, like *The Lancet*, was showing staying power with almost 13 years of unbroken publication by October 1840.[8] These first weeklies were all published in London and it is tempting to assume that they catered for a metropolitan audience. Wakley, despite his Devon origins, is alleged to have held provincials in contempt – though at first he had extended a warm welcome to the foundation of the Provincial Association.[9] We lack information on the regional distribution of the readership of *The Lancet* and its rivals. But examination of *The Lancet*'s pages reveals that it tackled provincial, Scottish, Irish and national topics, and that its correspondents resided in many localities. Green may have identified a 'gap in the market' for medical journalism, but it would be wrong to think that he was the first to try to reach provincial practitioners on a weekly basis. His best 'market opportunity' existed among PMSA members for, while the Association aimed to cultivate medical science and professional fellowship in the provinces, it had few means of so doing. Beyond the annual meetings, *Transactions* and, in some regions, local branch activities, there was little to unify members in a sense of common purpose and endeavour.[10] A weekly journal promised to supply the deficiency. But, with *The Lancet* apparently catering for a provincial market, was there space for a rival publication? That there was owed much to the coolness, not to say antipathy, which developed between Wakley and the PMSA.

Wakley's initial enthusiasm for the Association soon gave way to disenchantment owing to its reluctance to espouse the cause of medical reform. When, in 1836 a prominent member of the PMSA, John Green Crosse, attacked the weekly medical press for coarseness and other journalistic misdemeanours (it was obvious that he had *The Lancet* in mind), the rift was complete. Thereafter *The Lancet* became an outspoken critic of the PMSA, so much so that members of the Association may have baulked at being subscribers.[11] Green, who surely knew all this, probably believed that his journal could be the beneficiary. Green's plans would hardly have endeared him to Wakley, for not only would the *PMSJ* offer direct competition to *The Lancet* but, by aligning it with the PMSA, Green was courting a body Wakley had grown to despise. Hence, even if the *PMSJ*'s launch was not a symptom of a rift between Green and Wakley, it must surely have caused one. In fact *The Lancet*, which regularly reviewed the medical press, ignored the *PMSJ* for years.

In order to improve his chances of support from PMSA members Green let it be known that he intended 'to advocate all those objects for which the Association was formed, and to demonstrate the possibility of aiding the efforts of the scattered members of the profession'.[12] Shrewdly, he asked that a member of the Association's Council should join him as co-editor. Council nominated Streeten who had previously written for both the *Midland Medical and Surgical Reporter* (a quarterly founded by Charles Hastings before the launch of the PMSA) and the Association's *Transactions*. It also pledged that PMSA members would use 'all endeavours' to ensure the success of the new journal.[13] Thus, from the outset, the *Journal* and the Association enjoyed close links even though the Association was not the proprietor.

Even with this link the success of the new journal was in doubt. In some respects 1840 was an inauspicious time for the launch of a commercial venture, for the country was in the middle of the 'grimmest' economic slump of the nineteenth century.[14] However, the prospects for success were improved by two developments: lower stamp duty on newspapers and the communications revolution. The reduction in newspaper stamp duty from 4 pence to 1 penny in 1836 provided a major fillip to newspaper production and circulation.[15] It allowed the *PMSJ*, as a stamped newspaper, to be issued at a price of 7 pence per copy (including postage) as against 10 pence. Almost as important was the growth of the railway network. In 1830 fewer than 100 miles of track were open to public use; by the end of 1844 the figure was 2,235 miles – with the years of maximum growth still to come. Birmingham, which, in 1836, was 11 hours from London by fastest coach (not the mail coach), was less than four hours away once the rail link was completed in 1838.[16] The penny post, which was introduced in January 1840, did not mean more economical dispatch for newspapers, since the existing stamp duty already allowed for postal distribution to any location at no extra cost. But in time improvement of the postal service, including the extensive use made of railways for carrying the mails, led to a more efficient and comprehensive service both for newspaper distribution and for information gathering.[17] Without these developments the launch of the *Provincial Journal* may still have occurred but its survival, which was long a matter of doubt anyway, would have been far less likely.

Once the *Journal* was 'up and running' the connection between it and the Association was rapidly consolidated. First, members were offered a discounted subscription rate; then, from 1842, the Association made cut price bulk purchases in order that the *Journal* could be sent, as it has been ever since, to all members as a benefit of membership. But the PMSA was still not the proprietor, merely the main customer. As such it was supplying most of the *Journal*'s income while possessing no managerial and little editorial control. Following repeated demands from the London publisher for higher payments, the PMSA 'hijacked' the *Journal* by transferring publication from London to Worcester and making Streeten sole editor. With this transfer the *Journal* became the first medical weekly to be published outside London. Thereafter, it was 'devoted entirely to the interests of the Provincial Medical and Surgical Association, and published under the controul [*sic*] of its officers and council'.[18]

Presumably because the *Journal* was unprofitable, the Association's act of piracy – for such it surely was – was accepted without demur by its publisher. But Green not only objected, he demanded compensation. The PMSA Council eventually agreed to pay him more than £500 and called on members for donations. However, the results of this appeal were so miserable that Green's claim had to be met from the Association's coffers with the result that its accounts slipped into the 'red'. It was an inauspicious start to the PMSA's proprietorship. In many ways it foreshadowed the relationship between *Journal* and Association over the next two decades and more.

What became of Green after his link with the *Journal* was cut is unclear, though he certainly returned to Dublin for a time. He remained a member of the PMSA in 1849, but his name was absent from the following year's membership list. A possible last glimpse is provided in James Fernandez Clarke's autobiography:

> I may say that, some few years since, a man walked into the *Lancet* office in a state of apparently great destitution, and asked for some relief for pressing difficulties – difficulties of common maintenance. George Churchill [publisher of the *Lancet* and Wakley's 'factotum'] inquired what claim he had on the *Lancet*. I am 'Erinensis', he replied.[19]

The supplicant, having convinced Churchill of his identity by answering certain questions, received aid.

At first, PMSA members welcomed the opportunity to subscribe to a new medical periodical. 'This excellent weekly Journal' and 'a valuable acquisition – calculated to become a powerful aid to the interests of the association and of the profession generally' were among members' verdicts.[20] But no sooner had the Association taken over than reservations began to be expressed. One critic described it as being 'badly printed on bad paper, with bad ink, badly edited, and . . . badly folded'; another termed it 'effete . . . stale, flat and unprofitable'.[21] A notable opponent was William Budd, the epidemiologist. He thought the *Journal* too costly to produce, that it lacked quality and was generally surplus to the requirements of a body which met only once a year.[22] Others felt that it contained too much politics. Of course, the *Journal* always had its champions, but for two decades its existence was the subject of regular debate and repeated investigation. At times the opposition was so fierce that not only the *Journal*'s days, but those of the Association, seemed numbered.

The *Journal*'s cause was not helped by the rapid turnover of editors. Since 1870 it has had only six (seven from April 1991); during its first 30 years, however, it experienced nine quickfire editorial regimes.[23] Superficially these early editors left the *Journal* for a variety of reasons. After Green had been unceremoniously dumped, Streeten died in office in 1849. William Harcourt Ranking and John Walsh (who were joint editors) resigned, one after the other, in 1852 over plans to return the *Journal* to London. When London publication resumed in 1853 the new editor was the Scot, John Rose Cormack. He came with excellent credentials, having founded the *Edinburgh Monthly Journal of Medical Science* in 1841 and, on moving south, the *London Journal of Medicine.* On appointment he amalgamated the *London Journal* with the *PMSJ* under the title *Association Medical Journal.* Cormack survived for 33 stormy months during which time he became the first and last person to hold the posts of Association secretary and *Journal* editor. He resigned in 1855 when he had the secretaryship wrested from his grasp. Cormack's replacement was Andrew Wynter. After five years he left to pursue a literary career. His successor, William Markham, resigned in 1866 to become a Poor Law Inspector. Ernest Hart had two periods as editor. His first ended after little more than two years when he fell under suspicion of having embezzled BMA funds. He was succeeded by Jonathan Hutchinson who, as a medical practitioner was probably the most distinguished of all *BMJ* editors. He also occupied the editorial chair for the shortest period of all – less than a year – before resigning on grounds of ill health and pressure of work.

These early editors left the *Journal* for reasons which were apparently unrelated to their editorial performances. But there are grounds for questioning whether the official reasons for their departures always tell the complete story. Walsh, for example, while refusing to edit the *Journal* in London went on to become an outstanding London-based editor of the *Field* and author of 'the standard textbook' on shooting, *The Modern Sportsman's Gun and Rifle.*[24] Wynter's literary career was not a financial success; when he died in 1876 his widow was reduced to appealing through the *BMJ* for invalid boarders.[25] Markham, in becoming a Poor Law Inspector, was not realizing a long-cherished ambition for, at the time of his appointment he 'was not known to have ever been associated with any sanitary work, nor to have seen the inside of a workhouse in his life'.[26] Hutchinson's 'fragile' health actually held up for another 43 years; as he later said, what he most enjoyed about editing the *BMJ* was giving it up.[27] In reality, most of the early editors left because they could not stand the unremitting criticism to which they and their *Journal* were subjected by the Association's Council and members.

All this might suggest that the PMSA did not really want a *Journal*. Its founder, Charles Hastings, was certainly less than enthusiastic. When the Association 'ditched' the *Transactions* in 1854 he expressed regret that it rather than the *Journal*'s 'more ephemeral pages' were to close.[28] However, in principle, the Association did want a *Journal* of its own. After all, a weekly publication provided a far-flung membership, the majority of whom never attended annual meetings, with a tangible corporate identity. Not only could it do much for the recruitment and retention of members, it provided a weekly reminder that the guinea per year subscription did actually purchase something. Members could address each other in print; they could advance the status of the PMSA and of provincial medicine by publishing papers; and they could publicly express opinions on the questions of the day, such as medical reform or Poor Law medicine. As the president of the PMSA's south-western branch said in 1847, the *Journal* 'is the bond which keeps us together, the perpetual refresher of the feeling that we constitute one community, as well as the most valuable repository of the contributions of our members, and in a lower sense, the *quid pro quo*, which is most looked to as an equivalent pecuniary contribution'.[29]

On the other hand, there was a limit to what members were prepared to pay for these benefits. During the 1850s and 1860s up to 90 per cent of the Association's subscription income went on financing the *Journal*. To some it seemed that a *BMJ* 'tail' was wagging the BMA 'dog', that is, that the Association was becoming little more than 'a joint stock enterprise for the publication of a weekly journal which absorbs nearly the whole of the Association's income'.[30] Yet in many ways the early *Journal* was the Association; it was certainly its most visible part. As a result, many members appear to have assumed not only that they had an automatic right of access to its columns as contributors and critics, but also that they were justified in dictating the conduct of editorial business. These were the circumstances in which rapid editorial turnover occurred. In 1865 BMA members, at the end of yet another debate on whether to retain the *BMJ*, voted 'fairly and decisively . . . to have and maintain a journal'.[31] But similar votes of confidence had been given in the past. As it was, the performance of Ernest Hart, who was appointed editor in 1866, decided the issue. He possessed not only remarkable ability but the strength of character to overcome opposition. He more than anyone was responsible for transforming the *BMJ* from struggling obscurity into a glittering national and international success, with a huge readership, soaring reputation and substantial advertising revenue.

Hart, the son of a Jewish dentist, was born in Knightsbridge in or around 1835. He won prizes galore both at the City of London School and as a medical student at St Mary's. Although only 31 years of age when appointed to the *BMJ*, he had already made his mark as a medical journalist on *The Lancet*, playing a prominent role in that journal's famous campaign to reform metropolitan workhouse infirmaries (1865). With a break of 12 months in 1869–70 he edited the *BMJ* till his death in 1898. After his death Hart's second wife promised a biography, but no such volume ever appeared; as a result he is now a somewhat shadowy character shrouded by a wealth of ill-founded myth and rumour.[32]

Hart was a controversial figure of firm opinions. Argumentative, egocentric, intolerant, ambitious, clever and devious, his personality provoked strong reactions among those with whom he came into contact. He has been accused of murdering his first wife, who died in suspicious circumstances in 1861, of stealing more than £800 of BMA funds and of using the *BMJ*'s pages to advertise a bottled water in which he had a financial interest. He has been called a 'scoundrel', a 'beast', a 'swine', a 'rascal' and a 'skunk'.[33] During his second editorial term there were at least two attempts to sack him; once over alleged misconduct in the Emperor Frederick/Morrell Mackenzie affair, and once for appointing an unqualified nephew to his editorial staff. Some disliked Hart personally, while others could not stomach his uncompromising views on such controversial questions as compulsory vaccination. In 1885, when he stood (unsuccessfully) for election to Parliament as a 'radical' candidate, his Mile End constituency was flooded with anti-vivisection and anti-vaccination opponents.[34] But some of the antipathy he aroused was pure anti-Semitism. Hence, one anti-vivisectionist opponent, Charles Adams, wrote, with rather disparaging implications for the *BMJ*:

> To have pushed such a paper into such a position is a feat of which any press-man might well be proud, a feat which would hardly have been within the compass of any who had not in his veins the blood of that pre-eminently pushing race.[35]

'Pushing' was a word frequently used in connection with Hart. Even those who admired him recognized his faults. For example, Robert Farquharson, who succeeded him as chairman of the BMA's influential Parliamentary Bills Committee, called Hart 'a wonderful man, who would have come to the top in any position, and who, I think, deserved to be called a genius'. But, recalling Hart's habit of 'claiming the credit for everything which went right', Farquharson felt there were good reasons for his unpopularity.[36]

It seems certain that thwarted ambition led to Hart's departure from *The Lancet* in 1866, possibly after coming to blows with the editor, James Wakley. The occasion of this dispute was Hart's insistence on promotion to an assistant editorship and Wakley's equally insistent refusal. Following his departure, Hart retaliated by spreading the story that he had been *The Lancet*'s co-editor. This inaccuracy rankled sufficiently for *The Lancet* formally to refute the claim in Hart's obituary notice more than 30 years later. According to Squire Sprigge, a later editor of *The Lancet*, the circumstances of Hart's departure from that journal meant that he and James Wakley lived for years 'on terms of open hatred'. Hart would not have minded this, for he regarded the possession of enemies as a mark of journalistic credibility. As he told an American audience in 1893: 'An editor needs and must have enemies; he cannot do without them. Woe be unto the journalist of whom all men say good things'.[37]

Whatever one thinks of Hart, it has to be admitted that his abrasive personality was a two-edged sword. It made him unpopular, but it proved invaluable in his journalism, especially the campaigning journalism for which he made the *BMJ* justly famous. When Hart saw a good story he pursued it relentlessly, careless of expense or the opinions of those for whom he had no respect. Take the *Journal*'s role in publicizing the discovery of X-rays and their clinical potential.

Although a sick man with barely two years to live when news of Roentgen's discovery reached England in January 1896, Hart, recognizing the importance of the 'new photography', as it was called, appointed a young scientist, Sydney Rowland as the *BMJ*'s special commissioner on X-rays. Over a period of some 18 months Rowland produced a total of 17 articles, some superbly illustrated, of which 13 appeared in the first half of 1896. In the words of a historian of the early years of British radiology, the *BMJ* was turned into 'a journal of radiology in miniature' and as such provided invaluable publicity for the infant science.[38]

Journalistically and scientifically this foray proved a triumphant success; but what did it do for Hart and Rowland? Rowland happened to be Hart's medically unqualified (though highly able) nephew to whose appointment the BMA was loth to agree. When Hart objected, forcibly and characteristically, on the grounds that he wanted staff on whose 'personal devotion' he could count, and that he was in a position to appoint whomsoever he pleased to his staff, the Journal and Finance Committee, the BMA body which supervised *BMJ* activities, agreed to climb down, but also to investigate ways 'of facilitating the resignation of Mr. Hart'. As for Rowland, he was reprimanded for purchasing, at the BMA's expense, the X-ray equipment he needed for his work as commissioner. Rowland was sacked by the BMA less than a year after the death of his uncle.[39]

High among Hart's many achievements was the raising of *Journal* circulation and, as a consequence, of its advertising revenue. The additional income not only kept the *BMJ* alive but did much to pull the BMA away from potential financial ruin. Hart accomplished this not by going 'downmarket' but by producing a publication of outstanding scientific, clinical and literary merit as well as considerable political influence. He always believed, as he wrote soon after he became editor, that if the Association were to publish a journal at all it

> should not be inferior in the freshness and variety of its professional news – in its external influence in medico-social; medico-political and sanitary questions – in the extent of its circulation – its grasp of all the professional subjects which arise and its general acceptance in the Profession to any private enterprise.[40]

This suggests that Hart saw his task as being to challenge *The Lancet*'s position as leading medical weekly. Probably he was motivated in part by a desire to teach Wakley a lesson by reminding *The Lancet* of what it had lost by letting him go. Hart's difficulty was lack of money to finance the drive for excellence, for he considered the £600 pa that was available for literary and editorial purposes to be 'entirely inadequate' to allow the *BMJ* to compete effectively with its rivals. So he planned, by using his literary connections, his 'skill and experience in editing' and his business management ability to increase the *Journal*'s appeal, thereby raising its circulation and, in consequence, its advertising revenue. This would enable him further to develop its 'excellence and reputation'. He realized that additional investment would be necessary if the plan was to get off the ground, but so confident was he in his own abilities that he was prepared to underwrite any losses from his own pocket.[41]

It was a high risk strategy but one which worked brilliantly. Circulation soared. In 1867, after 26 years of publication, this stood at around 2500 per week with an annual rate of increase of around 40. When Hart took over, annual growth leapt to about 500. *The Lancet*'s circulation was surpassed in the early 1870s. By 1884 Hart was claiming a circulation greater than that of all the *BMJ*'s rivals combined and by 1886 a sale which exceeded that of its nearest rival by more than 250,000 per annum. At the end of the Hart era, circulation exceeded 21,000 per week, making the *Journal* the world's highest circulation medical periodical.[42]

As Hart had anticipated, advertising income grew alongside circulation. As early as mid-1868 he was able to report that this had quadrupled (from £500 to £2000 pa) since he took over.[43] Before Hart died, *BMJ* advertising and sales revenue were in some years providing a higher share of BMA income than subscriptions. This was partly because advertising rates were increased but mainly because the space devoted to advertisements was dramatically expanded. By 1899 the *BMJ* carried 64 pages of editorial matter but a staggering 80 pages of advertising. Advertising revenue saved the *Journal* and helped provide the launching pad for the BMA to become a wealthy and powerful interest group, occupying increasingly prestigious premises and stalking the corridors of power in Whitehall and Westminster.

The simplest explanation for the *BMJ*'s success under Hart is the high quality of its journalism. As soon as he was appointed Hart began a thorough overhaul of its contents. Before his arrival its pages had been dominated by reports of BMA business, particularly reports of national and local meetings plus a selection of the (often less than riveting) papers read before them. Hart reduced this material, placing far more emphasis on 'original communications', including scientific papers and medical news. Until his editorship the *BMJ* had an undistinguished record in publishing scientific and clinical papers by the leaders of the profession. *The Lancet*'s achievements in this area were far superior. Hart changed this, publishing papers by such luminaries as Joseph Clover, William Gowers, Robert Lawson Tait, Joseph Lister, Thomas Spencer Wells, William Osler, Patrick Manson and Ronald Ross. It is probably true to say that in the sixty years following Hart's initial appointment more major innovations in British medicine were first reported in the *BMJ* than anywhere else. Hart also began to aim the *Journal* directly at specific medical interest groups such as army and navy surgeons, Poor Law medical officers and regional practitioners in Scotland and Ireland – all of whom were given their own columns. Another thing he did was to develop the *BMJ* as a socio-medical journal. *The Lancet*, with its famous 'commissions' on such subjects as food and drink adulteration and workhouse infirmaries, had led the way in this area. But Hart, with his campaigns on baby farming, the contagious diseases acts and other issues, made the *BMJ* preeminent in the field.

These developments necessitated considerable change in the way in which the *BMJ* was assembled. There is little information about the manner in which the early editors put the *Journal* together, but, apart from the ubiquitous 'Association News' they seem to have relied heavily upon unsolicited items from BMA members, such as letters and case notes; reprinting lectures and the reports of learned societies; and recycling material from other journals. Probably they wrote many of their own leading articles. As critics frequently pointed out, the resulting mixture was not particularly exciting. The richly diverse and far larger *BMJ* produced by Hart had to be compiled in a rather different manner. Instead of relying on a permanent full-time staff of 'writers of all work', which Hart claimed was the habit of his rivals, he gradually established a large team of contributors on whom he could call for occasional or regular articles. By 1875 the *Journal* had part-time reporters in Edinburgh, Dublin, Liverpool 'and other great cities'. It also employed three men to cover the meetings of the London medical societies. Special correspondents covered overseas events such as medical congresses or wars. Hart himself visited north-eastern France in order to report on medical aspects of the Franco-Prussian War. By 1889 there were 'upwards of 140 members of the editorial staff', that is, regular contributors paid at a rate of 15 shillings per column, of whom between 30 and 40 contributed to any one issue. Six years later the editorial staff had grown to 250 including overseas correspondents.

Although Hart's changes did not give universal satisfaction – there were, for example, regular complaints that he gave insufficient attention to BMA branch activities – they do seem to have elicited a generally favourable response. It would be simplistic to credit Hart alone for the *BMJ*'s increased circulation. The late-Victorian growth of the medical profession and the constitutional link with the Association were more fundamental factors. But by producing a *Journal* of high quality and broad interest, Hart put the *BMJ* in a good position to capture a large slice of the growing market for medical journalism. It is, anyway, insufficient to suppose that the *Journal* was merely a beneficiary of the BMA's success. A case can be made for the reverse, for many BMA members were recruited after having first been *BMJ* subscribers.[44] Since membership of the BMA was (deliberately) cheaper than an annual subscription to the *Journal*, it was in the financial interests of those who wanted the *Journal* but who were not particularly interested in BMA membership, to join the Association anyway. In fact, under Hart the *BMJ* was systematically and successfully employed to recruit BMA members. For example, non-member non-subscribers who were in the profession were sent a free copy of the *Journal* every year in the hope that they would wish to obtain it regularly; non-member subscribers were offered a rebate on their subscriptions if they converted to membership. As the BMA's council observed in 1868: 'the character of the JOURNAL under the editorship of that gentleman [Hart] has been greatly instrumental in adding to the numbers and influence of the Association'.[45]

In time the lesson was learned in the United States. Like the PMSA the American Medical Association, which was founded in 1847, had published annual *Transactions* rather than a weekly journal. But the AMA continued with this for far longer than its British counterpart. In 1880, with membership figures stagnant, it was looking for ways of attracting new recruits. Lewis Sayre, in the course of delivering that year's presidential address, attributed what he called the 'conspicuous progress' of the BMA to the success of its journal under its 'accomplished editor', Hart. He suggested that the AMA should establish a weekly journal of its own. Three years later, following further recognition of the achievements of Hart and the *BMJ*, the *Journal of the American Medical Association* was launched. It was a transatlantic clone of the *BMJ*, planned with the explicit objectives of recruiting members for the Association, extending its influence and generating advertising revenue. Hence, the example of Hart's *BMJ* was directly responsible for *JAMA*'s appearance.[46]

Of course, it was one thing to improve the standard of the *BMJ* for a short time, but quite another to go on improving it and to maintain that improvement for years and decades. Yet Hart did this over a period of some 30 years. He also left the *Journal* well provided with a successor. This was Dawson Williams, who had been a contributor since 1881, and whom Hart had appointed a member of the editorial staff in 1886. Since this time, up to and including the 1991 change, the editorship has always been filled by internal promotion rather than by external recruitment.

In his interests, temperament and appearance Williams was very different from Hart. But when he became editor of the *Journal* he made no dramatic alterations, adhering instead to Hart's proven formula and introducing change only gradually. Circulation, which increased steadily, had reached 37,850 per week by the time Williams retired in 1928. Advertising and sales income also showed healthy growth; in 1928 annual revenue from these sources exceeded £58,300. Although this meant that the *Journal* invariably needed a subvention from BMA funds to cover costs, it did not mean that the *BMJ* was a loss maker, for the great bulk of its print run continued to go to BMA members as a benefit of membership. In contrast to the AMA, no portion of BMA subscriptions has ever been earmarked for the publication of a journal. By the same token, it is insufficient to evaluate the *BMJ*'s success in terms of increased circulation or revenue.

In terms of *Journal* content Williams placed less emphasis than Hart on medical politics and socio-medical campaigns. The national insurance struggle of 1911–1913 was fought not by the *BMJ* but by the Association. Even so, it was during his period as editor that the *BMJ* conducted its famous 'war' against secret remedies or proprietary medicines. But Williams's main interest was to develop the *Journal*'s status as a publisher of papers on medical science and clinical practice. 'Post-graduation training brought to the practitioner's door' was how he often described the *Journal*. William Gowers, Victor Horsley, Patrick Manson, William Leishmann and Almroth Wright were among the distinguished figures who published seminal papers in Williams's *BMJ* which, during the Edwardian years, was probably at the peak of its standing as a scientific journal. However, just as Hart's interest in political and social questions had antagonized some of his readership, so his successor's emphasis on science alienated others. Over-specialization and neglect of GPs were among the criticisms uncovered by a BMA committee, along with the suggestion that the editor should follow 'a course of "live" American journalism'.[47]

If Williams had resigned as editor at the end of the First World War, when aged 64 (already older than Hart had been when he died), he would now be regarded as having been an almost unqualified success. As it was, he stayed on for almost ten years longer, during which time the *Journal*'s reputation began to slide. Never in robust health, Williams suffered serious injuries when in a road traffic accident near Horsham in 1910; in 1920, when heart disease was diagnosed, he was given only weeks to live. Although he lived for another 8 years, his health, energy and judgement were impaired. Fearful of how he would spend his retirement, Williams clung to office until prised from it, in January 1928, little more than a month before his death, by the liberal financial inducements offered by the BMA. The experience persuaded the Association to introduce a mandatory retirement age of 65 for *BMJ* editors.[48] So when Gerald Horner took over he found 'the great journal . . . in a shaky condition'.[49] A dynamic editor was needed to spark a revival. But, unlike Hart, Williams had groomed no suitable successor. Horner, in fact, was quite unsuited to the task which faced him; assuming charge of an ailing publication, he unerringly piloted it into further difficulties.

Between 1911 and 1915, when he took a temporary commission in the RAMC, Horner had been an assistant editor on *The Lancet*. He was appointed to the *BMJ* in 1917 in circumstances which reveal much about the man. Hearing that Williams's assistant editor was planning to resign, 'Mrs Horner went of her own accord to see Dr. Williams, told him that Horner did not want to return to *The Lancet*, where he had already been replaced, and persuaded him to get Horner released from the army for the *B.M.J.*'.[50] Though, reputedly, kindly, courteous and knowledgeable, Horner was incapable of providing leadership, distrustful of innovation and lacking in confidence. In Squire Sprigge (at *The Lancet*) and Dawson Williams, Horner had worked with two of the greatest medical editors of the twentieth century. But far from being a source of strength, this pedigree proved a handicap for, having worshipped Williams he found it impossible to make changes in the *Journal*. As a result it became firmly 'stuck in a rut'. As his successor, Hugh Clegg, later recalled, the *Journal* 'wasn't being edited and people . . . [began] . . . to complain'. Important aspects of inter-war health and medicine, for example the relationship between health and poverty, were ignored almost completely. Horner, apparently, was more interested in matters syntactical.[51]

In some respects, notably in terms of its circulation and income, Horner's *BMJ* flourished. By 1939 circulation was almost 43,000 per week, while income (still chiefly from advertising) exceeded £70,000 per year. On the other hand sales to non-members – perhaps a better indicator of success given the *Journal*'s 'captive audience' of BMA members – were lower in 1939 than they had been in 1918. In 1938 the subvention from BMA funds to *Journal* coffers was higher than ever before. The Second World War brought significant gains for the *BMJ* in terms of higher circulation (as BMA membership grew) and (almost unheard of) financial surpluses as advertising rates were raised. Wars always supply medical journals with good 'copy', and the simultaneous planning of a National Health Service provided the *BMJ* with a long-running saga, of extraordinary interest to the whole profession, on which it was uniquely placed to report and reflect on the BMA's contribution. As a result, the *Journal* emerged from the war, in all respects in rude health. Whether Horner, who retired at the end of 1946, deserves credit for seizing the opportunities with which the *Journal* was presented is doubtful, for his eventual successor, Hugh Clegg, had *de facto* control perhaps from as early as 1939.[52]

Clegg, a pugnacious and unpredictable man, could hardly have been more different from Horner. He is often remembered for two acts of combativeness: first, defying the government ban on periodical publishing during the energy crisis of 1947 and, second, upholding editorial independence during the gold-headed cane controversy of 1956.[53] But in 1948, by using the *Journal* to restrain 'last-ditchers' in the BMA from refusing service in the NHS, he also accomplished a notable feat of reconciliation. In addition, he re-established both the *BMJ*'s interest in the social and political context of medicine and its standing as a publisher of original papers. Overall he did much to reverse the long-term decline in the *BMJ*'s reputation. It is true that he was the beneficiary of the *Journal*'s business success which, in the 1950s and 1960s, regularly yielded healthy financial surpluses – nearly £72,000 in the peak year of 1953. But these large sums were of little real value to the *Journal* since they passed straight into BMA coffers. Not the least of Clegg's achievements was to negotiate the retention of a portion of these surpluses for *BMJ* purposes, thereby ensuring the *Journal* more economic independence than it had ever before possessed.

When Clegg retired in 1965 he had achieved much. From the perspective of the 1990s the *BMJ* of the early sixties, with its absence of humour, close-printed columns, lack of colour and formal celebration of Royal anniversaries seems not only dated but somewhat narrow and austere. Yet Clegg may in time be seen as the editor who steered it towards a second 'golden age'. After 150 years its prospects call to mind Ernest Hart's response to a suggestion that his days as editor were numbered: 'here I am', he said, 'and here I mean to stay'.[54]

Notes

1. *Journal*, 13 June 1849, 319.
2. George D. Burtchaell and Thomas Ulick Sadleir (eds), *Alumni Dublinensis. A Register of the Students, Graduates, Professors and Provosts of Trinity College in the University of Dublin (1593–1860)*, Dublin, Alex. Thom, 1935, pp. viii–ix, 343; BMA mss. PMSA Minutes, 1834–47, Proceedings of the PMSA, Ninth Anniversary Meeting, York 1841. Report of Council.
3. Martin Fallon (ed), *The Sketches of Erinensis. Selections of Irish Medical Satire, 1824–36*, London, Skilton & Shaw, 1979, p. 8; J.F. Clarke, *Autobiographical Recollections of the Medical Profession*, London, Churchill, 1874, pp. 150–1; see Alexander Macalister, *James Macartney. A Memoir*, London, Hodder & Stoughton, 1900, p. 186; J.D.H. Widdess, *A History of the Royal College of Surgeons in Ireland and its Medical School, 1784–1984*, 3rd ed., Dublin, RCSI, 1984, p. 53.
4. Sir Charles Cameron, *History of the Royal College of Surgeons in Ireland and of the Irish Schools of Medicine; including Numerous Biographical Sketches; also a Medical Bibliography*, Dublin, Fannin, 1886, p. 339.

5. Fallon, op. cit., note 3 above, p. 9; *Lancet*, 8 Sept. 1838, 834–6; 15 Sept. 1838, 873–7; 1 June 1839, 380; 2 May 1840, 183–5.

6. *Journal*, 3 Oct. 1840, 1.

7. BMA mss., op. cit., note 2 above.

8. See W.R. LeFanu, *British Periodicals of Medicine, 1640–1899*, Oxford, Wellcome Unit for the History of Medicine, 1984.

9. Irvine Loudon, *Medical Care and the General Practitioner 1750–1850*, Oxford, Clarendon Press, 1986, pp. 280–1.

10. BMA mss., op. cit., note 2 above.

11. *Lancet*, 30 July 1836, 608–10; 12 Nov. 1836, 265; 31 Dec. 1836, 500–1; 15 July 1837, 593–4; 29 July 1837, 670–2; 5 Aug. 1837, 697.

12. *Journal*, 13 June 1849, 319.

13. ibid.

14. J.F.C. Harrison, *The Early Victorians 1832–51*, London, Weidenfeld & Nicolson, 1971, p. 12.

15. J.H. Wiener, *The War of the Unstamped. The Movement to Repeal the British Newspaper Tax, 1830–36*, Ithaca and London, Cornell University Press, 1969; W.H. Brock and A.J. Meadows, *The Lamp of Learning: Taylor and Francis and the Development of Science Publishing*, London and Philadelphia, Taylor & Francis, 1984, pp. 93–4; Howard Robinson, *Britain's Post Office*, London, Oxford University Press, 1953, p. 120.

16. J. Simmons, *The Railway in England and Wales, 1830–1914*, Leicester University Press, 1978, p. 271; H.G. Lewin, *The Railway Mania and its Aftermath, 1845–51*, London, Railway Gazette, 1936, p. 1; P.S. Bagwell, *The Transport Revolution from 1770*, London, Batsford, 1974, pp. 93, 129.

17. M.J. Daunton, *Royal Mail. The Post Office Since 1840*, London, Athlone Press, 1985, p. 10 and ch. 2.

18. *Journal*, 3 April 1844, 11.

19. Clarke, op. cit., note 3 above, pp. 151–2.

20. *Journal*, 31 Oct. 1840, 92; 13 Feb. 1841, 336; 25 June 1842, 236–7; 9 July 1842, 277; 16 July 1842, 288; 5 Aug. 1843, 379, 381; 5 Jan. 1856, 13.

21. ibid., 8 Aug. 1849, 429; 4 Aug. 1852, 397.

22. ibid., 14 Aug. 1844, 311; 10 Dec. 1845, 727–8; 8 Aug. 1849, 429.

23. The details are: Green and Streeten, 1840–44; Streeten, 1844–49; Ranking and Walsh, 1849–52; Walsh, 1852; Cormack, 1853–55; Wynter, 1855–60; Markham, 1860–66; Hart, 1867–69; Hutchinson, 1869–70.

24. R.N. Rose, *The Field 1853–1953. A Centenary History*, London, Michael Joseph, 1953, pp. 73–84; I.M. Crudgington and D.J. Baker, *The British Shotgun vol. II, 1871–90*, Southampton, Ashford, 1989; Hereford and Worcester Record Office, Foley Scrapbook vol. III, 82.

25. *Journal*, 20 May 1876, 637–8; 15 July 1876, 84.

26. Joseph Rogers, *Reminiscences of a Workhouse Medical Officer*, London, Fisher Unwin, 1889, p. 57.

27. *Journal*, 19 Aug. 1876, 231.

28. ibid., 27 Oct. 1854, 973–4.

29. ibid., 25 Aug. 1847, 466.

30. ibid., 1 July 1871, 20.

31. ibid., 2 Sept. 1865, 236–8.

32. See P.W.J. Bartrip, *Mirror of Medicine. A History of the BMJ*, Oxford, Clarendon Press, 1990, pp. 63–8.

33. *BMJ* mss. Ernest Hart file, Letters from F.R. Fisher to E.M. Little, 18 April 1929, 28 May 1929, 21 June 1929; R. Scott Stevenson, *Goodbye Harley Street*, London, Christopher Johnson, 1954, pp. 85–6.

34. *East London Observer*, 28 Nov. 1885; Robert Farquharson, *In and Out of Parliament*, London, Williams & Norgate, 1911, p. 117.

35. Quoted in R.D. French, *Vivisection and Medical Science in Victorian Society*, Princeton University Press, 1975, p. 347.

36. Farquharson, op. cit., note 34 above, p. 117; H.O. Barnett, *Canon Barnett, His Life, Work and Friends*, London, John Murray, 1918, I, p. 148; *Practitioner*, Feb. 1898, LX: 117–18.

37. *Lancet*, 15 Jan. 1898, 193; 6 Oct. 1923, 723; *Jewish Chronicle*, 14 Jan. 1898; *Medical Press and Circular*, 12 Jan. 1898, 40; *Journal*, 1 July 1893, 20; Stevenson, op. cit., note 33 above, p. 86.

38. E.H. Burrows, *Pioneers and Early Years. A History of British Radiology*, St Anne, Alderney, Colophon, 1986; see R.F. Mould, *A History of X-Rays and Radium with a Chapter on Radiation Units: 1895–1937*, Sutton, IPC, 1980.

39. BMA mss. Minutes of Committees and Sub-Committees, VIII, Journal and Finance Committee, 20 Jan. 1897, 3607–8; 14 Feb. 1897, 3672–4; *Journal*, 17 March 1917, 375; *Lancet*, 7 April 1917, 552; Bartrip, op. cit., note 32 above, pp. 137–40.

40. BMA mss. Committee of Council Minute Book, 1868–75, copy of letter from Ernest Hart, dated 20 June 1868, pp. 8–13.

41. ibid.

42. *Journal*, 14 Dec. 1878, 881; 1 Jan. 1887, 22; 5 Jan. 1884, 21.

43. BMA mss., op. cit., note 40 above, p. 11.

44. *Journal*, 24 Feb. 1872, 216.

45. ibid., 8 Aug. 1868, 147; 13 Jan. 1872, 49; 10 Feb. 1872, 159; 5 Jan. 1884, 21.

46. Morris Fishbein, *A History of the American Medical Association 1847–1947*, Philadelphia and London, W.B. Saunders, 1947, pp. 100–7; Paul Vaughan, *Doctors' Commons. A Short History of the British Medical Association*, London, Heinemann, 1959, pp. 134–5.

47. BMA mss. Minutes of Council Committees and Sub-Committees, Journal Committee, 4 April 1917, 430–1.

48. R. Scott Stevenson, *In a Harley Street Mirror*, London, Christopher Johnson, 1951, p. 5; *Journal*, 21 Jan. 1928, 103; 3 March 1928, 361; 10 March 1928, 414–25; 13 March 1954, 648–9.

49. *BMJ* mss. Horner file, Personal Memoirs, handwritten notes, pp. 8–9.

50. Stevenson, op. cit., note 33 above, p. 88.

51. *BMJ* mss. Clegg file, Transcript of Richard Smith's interview with Hugh Clegg, Jan. 1982; author's interview with T.D.V. Swinscow, 9 Feb. 1989.

52. ibid.; *BMJ* Supplement, 2 Aug. 1947, 40; *Times*, 7 July 1983; *DNB, 1981–90*, Oxford University Press, forthcoming.

53. Bartrip, op. cit., note 32 above, ch. 11.

54. *Practitioner*, Feb. 1898, LX: 118.

8

The American Medical Association and its journal

Elizabeth Knoll

Political tensions about the goals of the American Medical Association, and their expression to the membership and the laity, have existed since the Association was founded in 1847. The most important is the tension between serving and self-serving. For all its publicly stated devotion to quality of medical care and protection of the public health, how energetically critical of physicians in the public interest is the AMA prepared to be? Even if one were not sceptical on principle about any powerful professional organization's claims to selflessness, one could find some illumination in the preamble to the AMA's original constitution. The Association's purposes are listed thus:

> for cultivating and advancing medical knowledge; for elevating the standard of medical education; for promoting the usefulness, honor, and interests of the medical profession; for enlightening and directing public opinion in regard to the duties, responsibilities, and requirements of medical men; for exciting and encouraging emulation and concert of action in the profession; and for facilitating and fostering friendly intercourse between those engaged in it.[1]

Four of the six clauses refer exclusively to advancing the interests, both social and political, of the medical profession. But that's not surprising: of course the AMA exists for its own sake. What's more interesting is that, for the first fifty or sixty years of its life, it was those first two clauses about advancing medical knowledge and improving medical education that were the Association's main preoccupations. As the profession coalesced, self-promotion and self-improvement seemed to converge.

A second tension within the AMA also seems more acute in the second half of the AMA's life than in the first half. What is the relation of the *Journal of the American Medical Association* to the AMA? Who is whose creature? For much of the period since the Second World War, and certainly since the forced retirement in 1949 of Morris Fishbein – the most famous, probably the most gifted, and certainly the most colourful editor *JAMA* ever had – *JAMA* has been little more than an AMA house organ. It was one AMA activity among many, and not the most effective or impressive AMA activity at that. As a medical journal compared with its competitors, for most of the post-war years it was 'the king of the throwaways', in one unkind but not unfair phrase. However, perhaps until the great post-war battles over national health insurance, when the AMA and Fishbein launched a campaign so successful that even now physicians who were not even born at the time refer to any form of compulsory government-funded health insurance as 'socialized medicine', it would have been more accurate to say that the most important and widely influential thing that the AMA did was publish *JAMA*.

Both the AMA and *JAMA* were consciously modelled on their British counterparts. As the idea of an American medical association was being discussed and enacted in the mid-1840s, the apparent success of the British Medical Association in advancing the dignity and usefulness of the profession was often noted. Forty years later, as the ill-organized and uninfluential association was struggling to find an alternative to its dull, rather expensive, usually delayed volumes of annual *Transactions*, committee chairmen and recent travellers to England observed that the *British Medical Journal* helped increase BMA membership and put money in BMA coffers. They spoke enviously of the energy and brilliance of Ernest Hart.[2]

But the AMA was a very American enterprise, created as a response to the particular conditions of the not-very-united states of the 1830s and 1840s, by ambitious young men of the new middle class. In these years, Washington DC was not much more than a village built on a swamp, the home for a weak central government in a decentralized and still very much a frontier society. The population was mostly rural; the culture was aggressively individualistic and democratic, suspicious of all élites and all claims to authority, including those of the learned professions, who were regarded (not without cause) as so many conspiracies against the layman. Perhaps in Philadelphia or New York City, where the Columbia University School of Physicians and Surgeons had been born from the King's College of Physicians and Surgeons after the Revolution, some established hierarchies of class and professional authority existed. But not in the more remote towns linked only by muddy roads, or springing up besides river ports (like Cincinnati) and Indian forts (like Chicago), or in the farm houses. Lacking a supporting tradition as well as reliable and demonstrable practical effectiveness (to which the pragmatic Americans would have responded), medical remedies, medical learning, and doctors did not inspire especial respect. 'Will you make your boy a pill-peddler?' a passing physician on horseback asked the father of Nathan Smith Davis, one of the founders of the AMA, in 1833. Farmer Davis, unimpressed, looked up from repairing his rail fence and answered that he'd be as good a 'tin-peddler' as anything else.[3]

Moreover, it was not clear who exactly the 'doctors' were. Patients dosed themselves with herbal remedies and patent medicines (many consisting largely of alcohol or opium), which were probably no less effective than heroic blood-letting, and were undoubtedly more appealing. Medical sects flourished – most notably homoeopathy and Thomsonianism, which emphasized the use of botanical remedies. Even 'regular' physicians' training varied widely. It consisted largely of apprenticeship to an older physician and might be supplemented by courses of lectures at a medical school. It could also include caring for the horses and doing household chores as well as helping in the consulting office. Medical schools existed – in fact, their number doubled between 1830 and 1845;[4] there were 42 by 1850.[5] Many were proprietary institutions, which for their (sometimes short) lives could turn a handsome profit. The competition between schools was intense, so the pressure was on to keep the curriculum short and easy, and the terms for graduation light. When Charles Eliot become president of Harvard in 1869 – over twenty years after the organization of the AMA – he tried to institute written examinations. The director of the medical school objected, arguing that a majority of his medical students could barely write.[6]

Moreover, no enforced external standards of licensure existed apart from these rather dubious degrees. One could call oneself a doctor and practise as such about as easily and as legally as one can now be a 'therapist' in California. Periodic attempts were made by state medical societies to elevate medical school standards, but they were half-hearted and unsuccessful. No state would venture beyond the others to impose firmer standards; their students could simply go to another state that would confer the MD degree after a year or so of two thirteen- or fifteen-week terms, or much less.

To improve medical education, then, what was needed was a *national* effort, and someone to organize it who was energetic enough to write hundreds of letters, eloquent enough to make them persuasive, strong-willed enough to keep fractious and mutually suspicious physicians in agreement on a single goal, and young enough not to realize that the National Medical Convention he wanted had already been shown to be 'impracticable, if not positively Utopian'.[7] The man who met these requirements, and who was responsible for the founding of the AMA and its continued life more than any other single individual, was Nathan Smith Davis, a delegate to the New York State Medical Society from the village of Binghamton, New York.

If Morris Fishbein has been the glittering Lucifer of the AMA sacred history, Nathan Davis has been its Moses, leading a contentious following out of ignominy and towards, if not into, the Promised Land of organization and influence. He was born in 1817 on a farm in upstate New York, which at that time was sufficiently remote for his father to have cleared the original forest from the land. (Admiring biographers and historians of the AMA like to point out that Davis was born in a log cabin, log cabins having about the same iconic status for Americans as mangers have for Christians.)[8] Thus he was less than thirty at the time the National Medical Convention of 1846 was organized. Despite the protests of older members of the New York State Medical Society that such a convention could not succeed, Davis's impassioned letter-writing campaign drew 80 delegates from medical societies and colleges of sixteen states to a convention at New York University in May of 1846.

The nascent AMA was an upstarts' organization, simultaneously determined on self-improvement and self-promotion. According to Davis, 'the Convention was composed of the younger, more active, and, perhaps, more ambitious members of the profession'.[9] This group did not represent the whole of the regular medical profession by any means. More than half the delegates were from the state of New York and only eleven medical colleges – one-third of those in the country – sent representatives.[10] Davis himself noted in his history of the AMA[11] that the leaders of the profession – academic physicians from New York, Boston and Philadelphia – were not there. The absences were not due solely to indifference. The reforming zeal of the letters written by Davis and his colleagues had seemed offensively arrogant to some recipients. In a widely reported speech, a well-known professor at New York University attacked the idea behind the convention as 'aristocratic' – as much a fighting word in Jacksonian America as 'élitist' is today.[12] Some societies and schools refused point-blank to attend.

If anything, these objections merely proved to Davis and his supporters the need for a permanent source of pressure for improved medical education – and, by implication, a more intellectually acute medical profession. The preparatory correspondence must have raised the question of a permanent organization, for on the second day of their meeting the delegates endorsed a resolution in favour of a national medical association, a 'uniform and elevated standard of requirements for the degree of MD' to be adopted by all medical schools, backed up by a solid preliminary education, and a shared code of ethics for the whole profession. Davis argued vehemently against having teaching and licensing in the same hands – a point which met less general agreement. Committees were formed and another meeting was scheduled for the next year.

It was at that meeting in Philadelphia, in May of 1847, that the AMA was officially formed. Officers were appointed, and committee reports on the requirements for the MD degree, on pre-medical education, on a proposed code of ethics, and on the union of teaching and licensing were read and debated. In the American spirit, and perhaps in memory of the accusations of aristocratic leanings hurled the year before, the convention made a great point of its strictly democratic organization (an aspect of its governance that the AMA continues to emphasize). All this democratic reforming energy ran high enough that by the end of the first morning's session a representative from Maryland offered an exasperated resolution that 'no gentleman shall be permitted to speak more than twice on the same proposition nor occupy more than fifteen minutes for speaking, without leave of the convention'. This resolution was promptly adopted, but only after 'fifteen minutes' was changed to 'ten minutes'.[13]

By the time it adjourned, the association had given itself a name, had stipulated guidelines for medical education (lengthening the curriculum from four months to six months, with a minimum of three years' study, three months' study of dissections, hospital internship, and a method for making sure that students actually attended lectures), and embarked on a battle against quackery, nostrums and patent medicines that led to campaigns for public health legislation and government licensure of physicians and pharmacists. From then on the AMA met every year. Apparently it was so wary of factionalism and excessive concentration of power that its officers served for only one year and meetings were never held in the same city two years in a row. Committees were formed, to look into and report on the state of medical specialties, from surgery to obstetrics, on medical education, on association publications, and – most interesting for our purposes here – on the medical literature.

The medical literature, primarily journals, was a prominent topic of worried discussion from the very first years of the AMA – not surprisingly, when one remembers how intellectually and socially isolated many of its members were from one another, and consequently how dependent they had to be on whatever medical papers were available. Dozens of them existed, thanks to the supportive advertising of the patent medicines and the supportive politics of the medical schools who could gain reputation by publishing their own journal for their own faculty.[14] The committee reports on the medical literature are full of complaints that have a familiar ring to today's medical journal editors: there are too many journals with too few good articles, too much cribbing of both good and bad from each other, too much irrelevance, too much inflated and pretentious writing (the signature style, as Cmiel's study of nineteenth-century American speech *Democratic Eloquence* reminds us, of the rising middle classes).

One committee complained in 1850 that in the whole of the previous year's piles of journals there were only two 'experimental memoirs' of any value. It says something about physicians' wide interests that one of these articles was on the action of poisons and the other on the nervous system of the alligator.[15]

Mixed in with all this general worry about the shoddiness of medical journals was some patriotic feeling that the American medical profession ought to create its own medical literature rather than be dependent on England's,[16] which was simultaneously revered and envied. By 1856 Nathan Davis, as chairman of the committee on the medical literature, was urging that more American articles and textbooks be used in teaching,[17] and by 1869 a new group was formed, the American Association of Medical Editors. Samuel Gross of Philadelphia, one of the prominent academic physicians who had joined the AMA by this time, and who had been urging a more Americanized medical literature for some years, suggested that the AMA *Transactions* be published, not as an annual volume, but in a monthly journal. But it was not until 1883 that the *Journal* was founded.

Until that time, the minutes of the AMA annual meetings, the various committee reports and the scientific papers read at the meeting were published in an annual volume of *Transactions.* Over the years the *Transactions* had proved unsatisfactory: they were badly edited, poorly printed and expensive, and usually appeared later than they were announced, despite the editors' constant pleas to authors to read and return their galley proofs promptly. The editors complained that some of the best material from the annual meetings, which by rights was theirs, appeared in other journals and newspapers before the *Transactions* could be published. In the jumble of medical newspapers and journals, with their eye-catching advertisements and highly opinionated editorials, the AMA *Transactions* went largely unread even by AMA members, let alone the rest of the profession. As many as 2000 unsold copies would have to be disposed of, at considerable cost to a small treasury.[18] If the committees on medical literature, as well as the committee on publications, complained about the quality of the contemporary medical literature, they did so from within a glass house.

Perhaps as much to the point, quotations from committee reports and presidential speeches suggest strongly that by the late 1870s and early 1880s the leaders of the AMA were looking for a way to strengthen the organization. Thirty years after its founding, it had relatively few practical accomplishments to show for itself. Outsiders complained that gourmandizing and sight-seeing took up a suspicious amount of the annual meeting time[19] and the grand ambitions enunciated between meals did not receive much deference. Journal editors were quick to comment sarcastically that

> notwithstanding the numerous reforms attempted, recommended and resolved on by repeated 'whereases' and reiterated at every successive meeting by high-sounding resolutions, and published in each volume of the Transactions, yet, in effectuating any one of these, . . . the efforts of the Association . . . have resulted in signal and utter failure.[20]

This particular comment dates from the mid-1850s, but little in later years would change a sceptical outsider's mind about the Association's pretensions.

In addition to increased membership and respect, the AMA needed money. Because it had no formal headquarters and no paid officers – even the salary of $1000 for the permanent secretary was felt in the early years to be too much of a strain on the treasury[21] – its expenses were relatively low, but so were its revenues, about $5000 a year. Dues were $5 a year, which entitled a member to attend meetings and receive the *Transactions*, but the dues were demanded irregularly and collected ineffectively. Official membership fluctuated widely but seems to have hovered around 2,000 – a small percentage of the roughly 50,000 'regular' physicians.[22]

Again the success of the *BMJ* was noted, this time in boosting the BMA's membership and income. According to the 1880 president of the AMA, the *BMJ* brought in something like $25,000 a year, allowing the BMA to extend its activities and still have a few thousand dollars left over at the end of the year.[23] Dr Joseph Warren of Massachusetts (a descendant of the Dr Joseph Warren who was an organizer of the Boston Tea Party and who apparently shared his ancestor's taste for independence) declared in 1881,

> I would, Mr. President and Fellows, that the American Medical Association had, in place of its ponderous annual publication, a weekly journal published under its own immediate auspices; and I would that at its head we had an editor with a vigor equal to that of Mr. Hart, that he might, with his editorial staff, stir all the dry and moldering members into a new life, and that he might infuse into

> them an interest and activity equal to or even greater than that which the British Association shows today.[24]

Financial anxiety, intellectual restlessness and patriotic competitiveness combined happily to inspire the membership to agree that a journal be founded. The redoubtable Nathan Davis, now chairman of the Board of Trustees, sent out a mailing of 40,000 describing the proposed new journal; he reported at the 1883 meeting that he had received some 2,000 promises of support, which in addition to the projected advertising revenue should support the publication cost. Bids had been received from various printers and, since one from Chicago was lowest, Chicago was recommended as the place of publication. (Since Davis himself had been a resident of Chicago for some thirty-five years, and since he became the editor-in-chief of the new journal, it would be in the finest Chicago tradition if there were more to this convenient coincidence than met the eye.)

The first issue of the *Journal of the American Medical Association* was published on 14 July 1883, a mere month after it was approved in principle by the annual meeting in June.[25] Clearly, Davis and his committee on publications were putting it together long before it was approved and Davis officially made editor. The *Journal* was to appear weekly as a benefit of membership; outside subscribers would be charged $6 a year – a fiscal incentive to join the AMA for only $5 a year. It would contain thirty-two pages of papers, addresses, editorial comment, correspondence and miscellaneous information (which meant abstracts of the most interesting reports from other journals). As a stab at cosmopolitanism, regular letters from London and Paris would be included. As it turned out, the *Journal* often published reports from further afield, describing the startlingly and impressively clean hospitals of Germany, for instance, or the picturesque old cities and learned medical scholars of Buda and Pest.

In organization as well as in editorial tone, the *Journal* showed the Association's reformist tendencies. Unlike other journals of the day, the Association's *Journal* would *not* include any advertising for proprietary, trade mark or patent medicines – that is, any medicines with secret ingredients. This policy, upheld fervently by Davis and other leaders of the Association, put *JAMA* at a considerable disadvantage in obtaining advertising. Reading between the lines of AMA minutes in later years, one has the impression that subsequent editors felt frustratingly hampered (not to mention impoverished) at being cut off from this very lucrative industry, which flourished throughout the nineteenth century and well into the twentieth. Hundreds of firms made fortunes from soothing remedies like Pierce's Pleasant Pellets, Radway's Ready Relief and Pink Pills for Pale People[26] and their advertisements were everywhere. Despite the loss of potential revenue from patent medicine advertising, and despite some editorial wavering under John Hamilton, the second editor, the Association stuck with its stringent ruling.

In any case, there were enough acceptable advertisements, enough subscribers and enough publishable material to get the young journal off the ground. By the end of 1883 between three and four thousand copies were being mailed out each week[27] and the revenues from the *Journal* put the Association comfortably in the black. By 1885 the AMA's annual income had gone up to $18,000 a year. Subscription levels grew too, although much more slowly. It took twelve years to reach 6,000; by 1898 the circulation of *JAMA* was about 11,270, while the membership of the AMA was somewhere around 8000 – still less than one-seventh of the medical population of the country.[28]

Editorially, what was the *Journal* like? For all the comparisons with the *BMJ* and the glowing predictions that some day the *Journal* of the AMA would have 'a future even more brilliant than its English brother',[29] in its early years *JAMA* was somewhat uneven. The *BMJ* itself had commented augustly, six months before the first issue appeared, that with so many lively journals now being published in America, 'the proposed medical journal of the American Medical Association, which lies still in the womb of time, will have much to do to hold its own'[30] and Davis himself had warned the annual meeting when he was made editor not to expect too much.[31] Probably *JAMA* was no worse than some of its dozens of counterparts, and a good deal better than others – those that were, in the dry words of one historian, 'unrestrained by considerations of ethics or scientific verification'.[32]

The *Journal of the American Medical Association* was not strikingly different from other journals of the time. It included Association news; long, often windy speeches by presidents of medical societies, often on the state of medical care; more energetically phrased editorials by Davis himself, usually attacks on shoddy education, quackery, impure foods and alcoholism (he had once edited a temperance journal); case reports; abstracts from other journals, often translated from the European journals that were probably inaccessible to rural readers and perhaps incomprehensible to many urban ones; brief book reviews; and entertainingly peculiar random anecdotes clearly used for filler. Like most of its counterparts, *JAMA* published very few reports of experiments, and, apart from the chatty letters from London or Paris, little news of developments in medical, physiological or bacteriological science. Questions of medical politics tended to be discussed in high-minded but somewhat vague terms. In this crowded market, journals regarded each other with competitive eyes and no great gentleness. The AMA's new journal, edited and published in the wilds of Chicago, came in for some criticism and ridicule from the East Coast.

Two characteristics may have distinguished *JAMA* from other medical journals of its time, or (a slightly different matter) make it particularly interesting to a late twentieth-century reader. First were its campaigns, which were very much those of the AMA, but now expressed to a wider audience than the attendants at an annual meeting. The unifying character of *JAMA* in the 1880s (after several attempts to retire from the editorship, Davis finally succeeded in January 1889) was given to it not by the quality or abundance of its medical reports, but by its repeated and energetic decrying of incompetence, inefficiency and corruption in medical education, medical (or quasi-medical) practice and the administration of public health in large cities. Newspaper accounts of tenement overcrowding, of epidemics among immigrants on filthy ships, or the selling of watered milk or rotting meat excited *JAMA*'s wrath. So did almost anything to do with alcohol, then as now the leading self-medication either in its honest form or disguised in a patent medicine.

In light of the present AMA's attitude towards governmental involvement in medicine, which wobbles between wary acceptance and open hostility, it is ironic to see how eagerly *JAMA* and the Association in the late nineteenth century sought governmental regulation of the medical profession and the public health at the local, state and federal levels. The *Journal* and the resolutions called for state boards of health, state licensure of physicians (which would mean, of course, exclusion of homoeopaths and other 'irregular' physicians) and regulation of the preparation and sales of food and medicine.

The other striking feature of *JAMA* in its first ten or fifteen years was its extreme self-consciousness. The AMA was preoccupied with the quality of medical literature from the beginning; several lengthy committee reports in the years before *JAMA* was founded reviewed American medical writing and tried to explain why it was, in general, so intellectually shallow and uneducated. So when the AMA began publishing its own journal, both the editors and the most active readers went in for self-analysis, self-criticism and self-improvement. As the years went by, the *Journal* contained less organizational information and more scientific and clinical material, to the point that by 1895 some readers felt that the *Journal* was now too advanced and that it ought to print less scientifically demanding articles to reach its readers.[33]

Although the *Journal* many have been scrambling for material when it began publishing, by 1899 enough manuscripts read at the annual meeting were rejected that the president objected in his speech, arguing that all manuscripts should be published to give the readers themselves the right to select the bad from the good.[34] Since the president of the AMA served for only one year, while the editor of *JAMA* was a permanent employee, and moreover until 1911 was also the general manager of the whole Association, it may be imagined that the editor could afford to ignore him. As one reads the minutes of the AMA meetings and follows the slow climb of *JAMA*'s subscriptions and the AMA membership, it becomes clear that the *Journal* is one of the main preoccupations of the Association, and is far and away its most successful undertaking.

The establishment of *JAMA*, in short, did more to foster the AMA's reputation than anything else in the nineteenth century.[35] When the Association finally acquired a permanent headquarters in Chicago in 1896, it seems it was largely because *JAMA* needed a permanent home. *JAMA* may have been the AMA's possession, but the tail wagged the dog.

Any articulate and confident editor dominates his own journal. What is striking is that for such a long time the editor of *JAMA* was also the most powerful single figure in the AMA. In the 1880s this was due partly to the fortuitous contrast between Nathan Davis's energy and egomania, and the dubious competence of the salaried permanent secretary. Having no headquarters and an annual change of officers, the editor was by default the most stable figure in the Association and, by having a weekly voice to the membership, inevitably the most prominent. The nineteenth- and early twentieth-century AMA was a reformist organization, although not a very effective or well-managed one. The dignified part was provided by the presidential addresses and the resolutions; the efficient part (insofar as there was an efficient part) was provided by the journal. Theodore Roosevelt's jovial comment on the United States presidency, that it was 'a bully pulpit', might have been echoed by editors of *JAMA*, and they pounded the pulpit forcefully. Almost all the ten editors who served for more than a year (there have been fourteen altogether) have been extremely strong-willed and enormously energetic. Two were also very durable. The Association's structure (or lack of it), and its comparative weakness as a political force, gave George Simmons and Morris Fishbein tremendous influence in their two successive twenty-five-year reigns between 1899 and 1949.

George Simmons was editor from 1899 to 1924, a period of great scientific advance in medicine and corresponding improvement in *JAMA* (which as one historian warns was 'a mirror, not a beacon'.[36]) He started many new editorial features, some of which exist to this day, such as Medical News and Questions and Answers. He added new emphases on new instrumentation and new discoveries, with something of a journalistic flair.[37] The person and position of permanent secretary having been dropped when he was made editor, Simmons was also general manager of the whole Association until 1911, which gave him enormous *de jure* as well as *de facto* influence – neither of which he seemed shy about using. A native of England who had somehow made his way to Lincoln, Nebraska, Simmons had acquired a taste for both reform movements and editing, as well as medicine. After running the *Nebraska Farmer* newspaper and leading a citizens' revolt against the political machine that dominated the rough frontier state, he was temperamentally well-suited as editor of *JAMA* to launch editorial campaigns against patent medicines, fraudulent advertising and proprietary medical schools. (Curiously, given the AMA's monopolistic opposition to homoeopathy, Simmons was himself the graduate of a homoeopathic medical school.[38])

Even when the positions of editor of *JAMA* and general manager of the AMA were finally separated, the editor remained at least equal in rank to the general manager (the structural ancestor of today's executive vice-president), for both were responsible only to the Board of Trustees. Simmons's drive and ability, coupled with the growth of specialty societies that emphasized the AMA's uniqueness as the organization for the general practitioner, helped the considerable growth of the journal and the AMA. In 1900, *JAMA* had 15,000 to 17,000 subscribers and the AMA about 9,000 members,[39] out of about 100,000 'regular' physicians. By about 1901 *JAMA*'s circulation finally exceeded that of the *BMJ*.[40]

So it was *JAMA* that put the AMA on the map in the 1880s, *JAMA* that kept it there into the first part of the twentieth century, and *JAMA* (along with its fellow specialty journals) that sustained the AMA financially until the end of the Second World War. Even now that substantial dues are received and the AMA owns a large chunk of downtown Chicago real estate, the journals are still its second-largest source of revenue. In the late 1940s, *JAMA* and the other AMA journals were the main – almost the only – source of AMA income, bringing in all but $243,000 of the net revenue of over $1,600,000. Over 70 per cent of the payroll went to people who worked for the editor,[41] who at that time was in charge of all AMA printing. It was as if the AMA until Fishbein's decline – which was a consequence of the bitter post-war fights over national health insurance – was primarily the publisher of a set of journals as well as a consumer magazine, and of the most influential medical journal in the United States.

Here, at the smoggy end of the twentieth century, the AMA is still the largest medical publisher in the world, measured by sheer number of pieces mailed. The Association also retains its academic justification, by supervising the accreditation of American medical schools and graduate medical education and continuing medical education programmes, and by being involved in promoting public knowledge about science, defending animal experimentation, and running many conferences on biomedical sciences and public health. This non-profit corporation looks to many eyes very much like a for-profit corporation, complete with lavish headquarters, substantial public relations and lobbying staff in Washington DC, and extremely well-paid executive officers.

Lobbying for the interests of the medical profession is now widely regarded, by AMA members and outsiders, as the AMA's chief function. The AMA has changed a good deal since Herbert Burrell, a professor of clinical surgery at Harvard Medical School who reorganized the teaching of surgery in Boston's hospitals, argued in his 1909 presidential address against politicking and the placement of a representative in Washington. Dr Burrell warned that 'The employment of one individual to serve as a lobbyist in Washington or elsewhere is a mistake; it is the adoption of trade union methods and will sooner or later bring the medical profession into discredit'.[42] By 1938, however, *Fortune* magazine was commenting on the transformation of the AMA 'from a mild academic body into a powerful trade association'.[43] This is certainly the way that the AMA continues to be perceived, not least in the academic world, where an AMA member is something of a curiosity. For the most part, there are no more presidents like Dr Burrell, or the two Mayo brothers, or Frank Billings (who joined William Rainey Harper at the University of Chicago to build up Chicago hospitals and medical institutes and reformed Chicago medicine almost single-handedly), or Abraham Jacobi – who was imprisoned in his youth for his part in the revolutions of 1848, who after making his way to Manchester and then New York became a professor at Columbia, the founder and first editor of the *American Journal of Pediatrics*, a public health campaigner, and, in 1912, the first and last Jewish president of the AMA. As the AMA's activities have changed since the Great Depression and the Second World War, the Association's officers have tended to be clinicians in private practice rather than academics, who have risen up through local medical societies. Consolidating the political power and maintaining the independence, prestige, and wealth of the medical profession have been the officers' main preoccupations. In this they have faithfully reflected the interests of the majority of the members.

All this brings us back to *JAMA* which, after its unfortunate recent past as a forgettably mediocre house organ, has increasingly become a major medical journal with by far the largest circulation of any journal in the world, thanks to its distribution to nearly 400,000 AMA members and its controlled-circulation foreign-language editions. The quality of its clinical and even basic scientific submissions and publications has been rising in the last several years; academic and research physicians who had barely heard of it ten years ago now subscribe. Although such readers might not join the AMA, the improved reputation of *JAMA* in this community is entirely to the benefit of the AMA and the AMA's reputation, as the governing hierarchy is well aware.

The moral and political tone that the journal has taken is another matter. In a striking break with his recent predecessors, the present editor, George Lundberg, strongly believes that a medical editor's job is to be the conscience of his profession. Since he became editor in 1983, many articles on professional questions – such as methods of cost control in medicine, the impact of regulation on medical care and costs, the number of 'impaired physicians' and means to treat them – as well as the many articles on public health, epidemiology and biomedical ethics have made *JAMA* more than 'merely' academic. Many of these articles challenge common assumptions of the politically conservative membership. Many of them, and many of the editorials written by the editor, criticize some features of the medical profession. They express determination to see it reformed from within, and this determination is expressed in unsubtle, fervent, multisyllabically moralistic language strongly reminiscent of the first editorials of *JAMA* a century ago. The intellectually imperialistic present editor of *JAMA* wants physicians to be moral leaders of the national community as well as skilful technicians; he calls on them to be as dedicated to the health of the public and of the body politic as they are to the health of their individual patients with paid-up insurance.

In this vision, Lundberg has more in common with Nathan Davis and his immediate followers than with any of his twentieth-century predecessors. Philosophically and rhetorically, he is a throwback to the AMA of the nineteenth century, which was spoken for by its *Journal*. The AMA of the late twentieth century is a different creature. It is much larger, much better fed, and perhaps much more frightened because it has so much more to lose from the suspicious hostility of the federal regulators and legislators on the one hand and the general public on the other. Observers must wait to see whether *JAMA* under Lundberg can be a strong enough tail to wag this big, anxious, angry dog into substantial self-criticism, and self-improvement. Many signs now suggest that the AMA is becoming a more representative, responsive and responsible organization, but the changes are slow and the signs are ambiguous.

It may well be, in the classic words of one of the late Mayor Daley's aldermen, that Chicago ain't ready for reform. If so, the relations between the AMA and its *Journal* – once its voice, now its more or less loyal opposition, but by far its best public relations tool in the world of academic prestige – will only become more interestingly strained. It is worth recalling that none of the editors of *JAMA* has resigned entirely voluntarily.

The history of the *Journal of the American Medical Association* is complex and rich; its longest and best version could be a window on the history of the AMA, the social history of American medicine, and perhaps even the well-intentioned, innocently self-serving, high-minded self-congratulation of professional organizations. The self-serving ideology is rightly exposed and criticized, but the high-mindedness, and its occasional genuinely publicly beneficial consequences, cannot be entirely dismissed. For the fullest and best history of the American Medical Association and its journal – as for any other history – all interpretive truths would be in nuance and emphasis, and in maintaining some generous fairness to the living and the dead. The best remedy for partial history is more thought, and more history. Nathan Davis once observed tartly that a common error in the medical and general literature

> consists in presenting the extravagencies, both in doctrines and practice, of each medical era, as evidence of the character of the medical men and practice of that time. Every age or generation has its extremists who become extravagant . . .; and their extravagancies are sure to be recorded on the pages of the current literature, and to be quoted by all subsequent generations as characteristic of that time. . . .

We can only agree with him that 'The only remedy for these popular and unjust errors is . . . an honest and thorough study of the history of medicine as a necessary branch of medical education'.[44]

Notes

1. Morris Fishbein, *A History of the American Medical Association*, Philadelphia: Saunders, 1947, p. 30.

2. ibid., p. 101.
3. Nathan Smith Davis III, 'Nathan Smith Davis, M.D., A.M., LL.D', in Fishbein, op. cit., note 1 above, p. 3. See also Paul Starr, *The Social Transformation of American Medicine*, New York: Basic Books, 1982, chapters 1 and 2, especially pp. 56–9, 82–5.
4. Fishbein, op. cit., note 1 above, p. 21.
5. Starr, op. cit., note 3 above, p. 42.
6. James G. Burrow, *AMA: Voice of American Medicine*, Baltimore: Johns Hopkins Press, 1963, p. 9.
7. Nathan Smith Davis, *History of the American Medical Association From Its Organization Up to January 1855, To Which is Appended, Biographical Notices, With Portraits of the Presidents of the Association, and Of the Author*, edited by S.W. Butler, Philadelphia: Lippincott, Grambo and Co., 1855, p. 23.
8. ibid. p. 184; N.S. Davis III, op. cit., note 3 above, p. 3.
9. Davis, op. cit., note 7 above, pp. 37–8.
10. Fishbein, op. cit., note 1 above, p. 26.
11. Davis, op. cit., note 7 above, p. 38.
12. See Kenneth Cmiel, *Democratic Eloquence: The Fight Over Popular Speech in Nineteenth Century America*, New York: William Morrow, 1990.
13. Fishbein, op. cit., note 1 above, p. 28.
14. ibid., p. 53.
15. ibid., p. 53
16. ibid., p. 32.
17. ibid., p. 60.
18. ibid., p. 88.
19. ibid., pp. 74–5.
20. ibid., p. 65.
21. ibid., p. 86.
22. Lester S. King, 'The founding of *JAMA*, 1883', *JAMA* 1983, 250: 179.
23. Fishbein, op. cit., note 1 above, p. 101.
24. ibid., p. 104.
25. King, op. cit., note 22 above, p. 177–80.
26. Burrow, op. cit., note 6 above, p. 70.
27. Fishbein, op. cit., note 1 above, p. 113.
28. King, op. cit., note 22 above, p. 180.
29. Connor, quoted in Fishbein, op. cit., note 1 above, p. 117.
30. Anonymous, 'Medical journals in America', *BMJ*, January 13, 1883, 68–9 (no volume number). I thank John Burnham for pointing out this reference to me.
31. Robert W. Riley, 'A century of editors', *JAMA* 1983, 250: 230.
32. Burrow, op. cit., note 6 above, p. 9.
33. Fishbein, op. cit., note 1 above, p. 172.
34. ibid., p. 193.
35. Burrow, op. cit., note 6 above, p. 13; King, op. cit., note 22 above, p. 180.
36. Lester S. King, personal communication, 30 October 1990.
37. Fishbein, op. cit., note 1 above, p. 196.
38. ibid., p. 350.

39. Burrow, op. cit., note 6 above, p. 13; Fishbein, op. cit., note 1 above, p. 199.

40. Frank Luther Mott, *A History of American Magazines Volume IV: 1885–1905*, Cambridge, Mass.: Harvard University Press, 1957; Fishbein, op. cit., note 1 above, pp. 199, 202.

41. Frank Campion, *The AMA and US Health Policy Since 1940*, Chicago: Chicago Review Press, 1984, pp. 113–14.

42. Fishbein, op. cit., note 1 above, p. 257.

43. Quoted in Mae Rudolph, 'When *JAMA* was king.' *MD*, 1990, 34: 51–61.

44. N.S. Davis, 'The basis of scientific medicine and the proper methods of investigation', *JAMA*, 1891, 16: 120.

9

The *British Medical Journal* in America

John Burnham

For 150 years, the *BMJ* has circulated all over the world. Yet the *British Medical Journal* and the predecessor *Association* and *Provincial Medical Journals* were based explicitly and institutionally in the medical culture of a geographic area. This accident of culture raises questions in the lively field of transnational, that is, transcultural, scientific communication – indeed, the whole field of the communication of knowledge and particularly medical knowledge. But I want to focus particularly on a related question that might tactlessly be phrased: how important was this institution, the *British Medical Journal*, not within the parochial confines of the UK, but in world medicine?

The three questions of cultural nationalism in medicine, scientific communication, and impact are not only interrelated but cannot be disentangled from one another. Nor can they all be addressed in a short paper. But I have made some casual samplings of the changing place of the *BMJ* in comparable journals of another national culture, that of the United States of America. And from such data, I hope, in a very rough way, to suggest the profile of the fate of the *BMJ* in the whole world of medical knowledge and institutions in the past century and a half.

Relations between the Anglo-American medical communities

Using any single national culture as a gauge naturally brings its own hazards, and the culture of the United States is no exception. It is customary to begin all discussions of Anglo–American cultural relations with the indignant reaction of nationalistic

Americans when, in 1820, the *Edinburgh Review* published Sydney Smith's sneering enquiry about cultural achievements in the United States: 'Who reads an American book?' he asked and, tellingly, 'What does the world yet owe to American physicians or surgeons?' The Americans' indignation was the greater because Smith was so largely correct in his contention that, intellectually, Americans were not independent or even very significant. In 1849, the editors of the *Provincial Medical and Surgical Journal* reprinted with obvious glee a lament from the *Transactions of the American Medical Association*, the author of which used an abundance of metaphors to say that, because medical journal editors copied so freely,

> The fairest fruits of British genius and research are shaken into the lap of the American student, and the great danger seems to be, that in place of the genuine culture of our own fields, the creative energy of the country shall manifest itself in generating a race of *curculios* [parasitic beetles] to revel in voracious indolence upon the products of a foreign soil![1]

For generations, well past the 1840s, medical as well as literary figures in the two countries traded insults across the Atlantic by way of the periodical literature; indeed, formal diplomatic relations suffered because a common language made it so easy to read inflammatory statements made by nationalists on either side. As late as 1870, a writer in the *Medical Times and Gazette* attacked American medical journals specifically: 'in America . . . the Medical newspaper exists only in the most rudimentary form . . . The average American medical journal is lamentably deficient from a scientific point of view; ordinarily it rests far too much on others, far too little on itself'. Even the writing was deficient, he continued, because of too much 'slanginess'.[2]

It was no wonder that Americans, still acutely aware of their continued colonial reliance upon British medicine and culture, countered with comments about 'haughty and arrogant' and condescending Britons. Yet by the end of the nineteenth century, the war of words had given way to considerable mutual respect; in 1883, an editorial writer in the *BMJ* claimed that 'the progress of American medical journalism in the last few years has been very remarkable', noting that the best American journals 'compare favourably with the medical journals of any country'. Most importantly for my concern, as the Bristol surgeon, J. Greig Smith, for example, pointed out in 1893, the better American medical writers were outstanding in the world for the thoroughness of their citations of scientific and clinical literature.[3]

In attempting to gauge the place of the *BMJ* in the medical literature of the United States, then, among a number of complications the most significant was the continuing change that took place in the role that American medicine, for its part, played in the world. Where at first American medicine continued to be colonial to that of Great Britain, later, particularly in the twentieth century, the former colonials began to export as well as import biomedical knowledge until the Colossus of North America rose to pre-eminence in biomedicine.

The *BMJ* itself offers evidence of this change. In a sample from 1903, out of 409 articles cited by *BMJ* authors, approximately 8.6 per cent were from American journals, compared to 11.0 per cent from French and 20.5 per cent from German-language journals. In that same time period, the *BMJ* carried 401 abstracts, mostly of non-British journal articles, and already approximately one-fourth were from United States journals and almost exactly the same proportion from French journals (26.9 per cent), while 34.2 per cent were from German-language serial publications. By 1923, out of 537 citations, *BMJ* authors took 24.9 per cent from American serial publications – but only 6.9 per cent from French and 15.3 per cent from German-language publications. In the abstracts, again the American and French were about one-quarter each, but the German-language items had diminished to 19.3 per cent. By 1953 (when there were no longer abstracts), American citations constituted 37.2 per cent of 1,472 in the *BMJ*, but French citations had dropped to only 1.6 per cent, while German-language articles (which included those from Austria and part of Switzerland) constituted but 4.3 per cent of those cited in the *BMJ* – altogether a dramatic demonstration of the Americans' rise in the world of medicine.[4]

As the unaccounted percentages suggest, *BMJ* authors tended on the whole to cite not foreign literature but writers out of the British medical community – a tendency common to all well-established medical communities and one of the evidences of the existence of national cultures in medicine. In the United

States, the tendency to cite only local articles eventually became far stronger than in Britain, so that by the 1980s, as measured by citations, the medical culture of the US had become anglophone and parochial to the point of scandal – which, again, meant that the United States presents a special test for the impact of an English-language medical journal.[5]

Mid twentieth-century evidences of the prominence of the BMJ

In addressing the question of the importance of the *BMJ* in the world at large, as opposed to the importance of the *BMJ* in Britain, I am attempting therefore to gauge how successfully the *BMJ* overcame the provincial resistances of other national medical cultures and penetrated into those cultures.[6] My focus is on the institutional functioning of medical journals and on the journal article. The convention of communicating knowledge by publishing journal articles, as John Ziman has pointed out, has been at the heart of the world of science for some time.[7]

That the *BMJ* was consistently one of the major medical periodicals of the world can be easily established. Since the 1930s, at least, those recommending journals for medical libraries, those compiling standard indexes, and those doing citation studies all agreed: the *BMJ* was a conspicuous and even essential medical journal.[8]

In the mid-twentieth century, a number of researchers, faced with the problems of librarians, investigators and clinicians trying to deal with a continually expanding number of scientific and medical journals and articles, began to publish selective lists suggesting which journals had the most use. Collectively these investigators showed that there existed essentially a hierarchy of publications: a very few journals, typically from 2 to 10 per cent, published the most utilized papers, typically 50 to 80 per cent of the use. At the same time, a very large number of papers, indeed, the bulk of the papers, had few or, perhaps, no readers other than the author (for the number of uncut pages in collections of reprints dating back many decades makes it doubtful that even the recipients of reprints necessarily added to the actual number of readers). Sometimes investigators tested how many journals were used in a library; sometimes they did a more or less sophisticated citation count.[9]

In all such compilations that appeared in the American and world literature of science and librarianship, I found that the *BMJ* was omitted from only two, both of which tried to use expert opinion to guide practitioner or hospital small libraries; but in those two cases of omission, the *Journal of the American Medical Association*, for example, was also not included consistently. Only *The Lancet* was almost universally present in such extremely selective lists as a token non-American item. But it should be emphasized that the two non-recommendations were aberrant; otherwise the *BMJ* did appear, consistently, right alongside *The Lancet* among titles suggested for library subscriptions. In the pioneer list assembled in 1937 by Jennie Gregory on the basis of citations in bibliographies, the *British Medical Journal* was tied for third place with the *Archives of Internal Medicine*, behind only *JAMA* and *Lancet*. The *BMJ* appeared also in later notable examples such as the standard list of journals for 'the small medical library' that first appeared in 1965 and in another, contemporary list issued by the American Medical Association.[10]

Altogether, such lists of recommendations based on samples of actual use and citation left no doubt of the high standing of the *BMJ* among experts from the 1930s on. Surveys showed consistently that any American library that would cover the top ten or twenty medical journals of the world, or would cover with a few titles even half or three-quarters of patrons' requests, would have had to subscribe to the *BMJ*.

The journals ratings game shifted away from the popularity poll model decisively and became much more intense in 1961 with the founding of *Science Citation Index* and the refinement of journal comparisons on the basis of how many times an article was cited. In 1972, the *BMJ* ranked twenty-seventh among all scientific (not just medical) publications in the world in the number of times papers in the journal were cited, and in 1987 (out of approximately 4,300 journals) it was still thirty-first, ahead of *JAMA* but behind the *New England Journal of Medicine* and *Lancet*, a relative standing within the medical realm that has not changed since the ranking began. Among general medical journals, the *BMJ* rated first in the factor of immediacy, that is, in number of recent papers cited.[11]

There was, then, in the middle and especially late twentieth century, substantial evidence of the place of the *BMJ* among scientific and biomedical journals. In the present paper I am attempting, by extending citation counts backward in time, to trace how the *BMJ* reached that high ranking.

Impressions and circulation figures

Beyond the citation counts, there are two other obvious kinds of evidence suggesting the impact of a journal, namely, circulation figures and impressions of knowledgeable people of the past. From earlier times, there are a few impressionistic indications of the status of the *BMJ* in the American medical community. In 1893, for example, the American Medical Editors' Association invited the editor of the *British Medical Journal* to address the group, in obvious recognition of the eminence of the journal, which had, after all, inspired a number of Americans to found *JAMA* in imitation of the British. And already in that period, Americans could report openly, that, in its class, the *BMJ* was 'king'. From a later period, to cite another example, Peter Bartrip quotes Walsh McDermott of Cornell Medical College, writing in the 1960s to retiring editor Clegg and referring to a perceived decline between the two world wars, 'When you started with the *BMJ* it really had relatively little influence on this side of the Atlantic, but under your leadership it has become a "must" for all of us here'.[12]

So far these impressions do not aggregate into a history, although they do give signs of reputation; this of course is not necessarily the same as influence, although when a high reputation became traditional, so that paying attention to a journal became customary, then influence was certainly involved. *The Lancet* benefited more as a traditionally leading journal, but clearly the *British Medical Journal* from the late nineteenth century was traditionally a powerful institution, and that factor alone meant that availability, custom and symbol made any paper in the journal more available and more likely to be cited.[13]

Circulation, beyond indicating at least potential readership, also added to the reputation of a journal. In 1909, for example, the prominent British physician, David Walsh, noted for an American audience the importance of the *BMJ* and went on to observe that the *British Medical Journal* of his day had 'probably the largest medical circulation in the world' (approximately 24,000). Even though in fact the *Journal of the American Medical*

Association (with 56,000 in 1912) already by then surpassed the *BMJ* in circulation, so much of the *JAMA* circulation was domestic that, in the world as such, Walsh was probably correct, and of course he introduced the circulation factor to bolster his impression. The importance of circulation, unfortunately, like impressions, can only be inferred. As late as 1940, the *BMJ* circulation was only about 43,000, compared with the 97,000 of *JAMA* in that year, but the citations (see below) suggest much more equality of impact.[14] (The *New England Journal of Medicine* at that point had only 6,600 subscribers, although by 1960 the circulation had grown to almost 60,000; in this case, too, the change in circulation was not fully reflected in citations; again, see below.) In the case of the *BMJ*, total circulation was to a large extent based on membership in the BMA, and therefore it was to some extent irrelevant to the reputation and influence of the journal. Moreover, for a variety of reasons, in the second half of the twentieth century, the circulation outside the UK declined in absolute numbers while the UK circulation almost doubled (from 48, 892 in 1960 to 83,683 in 1989). Circulation of the *BMJ* in the United States, by contrast, increased to about 1,800 copies in 1960 and levelled off at between 3,000 and 4,000 during the next thirty years – probably reflecting American research and library budgets (and the relative strength or weakness of the dollar) more than other factors.[15] Altogether, circulation figures are not very helpful in indicating how and why a journal had influence. In 1913, for example, almost 25 per cent of the subscribers to *Nature* were located in the United States – but *Nature* did not have an association base in the UK as did the *BMJ*. Moreover, the editors of *Nature* aspired to make it international in a way that was not appropriate for the organ of the British Medical Association, although the editors of the *BMJ*, too, aspired for international recognition, regardless of the circulation distribution.[16]

Changes in the phenomenon of citation

Given the difficulties of using circulation figures, counts of citation frequencies take on significant plausibility as a best first measure of the impact of the *British Medical Journal*. In setting up the study of citation frequency, I did have to take account of the fact that earlier data are not commensurable with those of the later period and specifically not commensurable with those derived from the *Science Citation Index*. First of all, as late as the 1840s, the convention of the reference had not yet developed in English-language medical periodicals, and many papers had none, either in the text or in footnotes or endnotes. Nevertheless, some comparable evidence is available from another convention which developed at that time and which allows counting, namely, the convention, to which I have already referred, of abstracting papers from other contemporary journals.[17] It is possible, therefore, to measure the presence of the *British Medical Journal* not only by examining references and bibliographies but, for earlier years, by calculating how many times an American editor or abstracter abstracted an item from the *BMJ*. Indeed, perhaps the first substantive citation of the *BMJ* in the United States was an abstract of a French article on resection of the elbow joint; the abstract appeared in the 31 March 1841 *Provincial Medical and Surgical Journal* and was reproduced – with credit – in the July 1841 *American Journal of the Medical Sciences*.[18]

In the last decades of the nineteenth century and the first decades of the twentieth century, the authors of original papers did increasingly take up the convention of citing references. For those decades, then, many journals contained both abstracts and references. Then by at least the period before the Second World War, the abstracts dropped out, just as they did from the *BMJ* itself, and references alone provide the basis for quantitative calculations of the flow of medical lore across the Atlantic.

From the 1840s, the *Provincial Medical Journal*, for its part, included abstracts of items from American medical periodicals. All internal evidence indicates that the chief source of the abstracts was numbers of American journals received in exchange, as was the custom then. That is, both producers and consumers believed that a journal should serve to a substantial extent to keep readers abreast of the larger world of medicine through reviews and abstracts, in addition to original contributions in the journal in article form. So in 1858 an American writer commended a British author for 'his diligence in finding out and displaying to his readers the researches and results of those actively engaged in scientific labours, in Germany and France as well as in England and our own country'. Since, as another American, R.H. Page, noted in 1879, few physicians were able to do research, it was the job of the editor to use his journal to inform his colleagues of useful or potentially useful knowledge and so act as 'a safe and sure director to the profession on its onward and upward course'.[19] It was to that end that editors of the nineteenth century exchanged copies of their journals for copies of other journals, and in this way, without the cost of a subscription or the need to haunt a library, an editor could have in hand a substantial amount of the medical literature of the day, which some staff member or associate could then summarize, or abstract, for the readers. In the practice of trans-Atlantic exchange, the editors of the *Provincial, Association* and *British Medical Journals* of the mid-nineteenth century drew their American abstracts almost exclusively from the *American Journal of the Medical Sciences*, the *New York Journal of Medicine, Transactions of the Philadelphia College of Physicians*, and one or two other publications. The journals which these early editors were exchanging, in short, were at least at first very limited in number.

Yet in their intellectual colonial dependency upon Britain, editors of medical publications in the United States gave a full measure of attention to journals published in the UK. A casual search of some nineteenth-century American medical journals, even local journals in which there was no evidence of an exchange with the *BMJ*, such as the *Ohio Medical and Surgical Journal*, turned up no instances in which, if there were abstracts or citations, the *BMJ* was not sometimes cited; indeed, in the interest of efficiency I had to abandon the search to find corners of American medical publishing into which the *BMJ* did *not* penetrate. Yet the sources of citations in obscure and local publications are a mystery, and it may be that, like most content of second-rate American journals of that period, they were lifted from other, more accessible American journals.

I base my scepticism upon one hard piece of evidence that numerically few Americans had access to copies of the *BMJ*, namely, the number of libraries in the United States that held runs of the *BMJ* as recorded in the mid-twentieth century *Union List of Serials*. Scholars and librarians continue to assume that *the bulk* of these sets, if not always originally in the listed library, were acquired in the United States and therefore reflect at least in part past subscriptions – since holders of a substantial run of a journal were unlikely to throw it out. There were in fact 16 partial or complete sets of the *Provincial Medical and Surgical Journal* (only four absolutely complete) and 19 sets of the

Association Medical Journal. (Canadian libraries, representing a somewhat different tradition, had only one and four copies, respectively.) More than 100 libraries held substantial runs of the *British Medical Journal,* 34 of them that began with the 1857 issues and an additional 35 that started before 1880, with a curious blip of runs beginning in 1877–78.

Lest one think that the 103 surviving runs of the *BMJ* were inconsiderable, or that the number in any way undermines a conclusion that even in the nineteenth century the *British Medical Journal* had an important presence in the United States, let me just note that the American medical periodical with the largest circulation in the 1870s, the *New York Medical Journal,* in the 1950s was represented in major historical runs in only about 67 libraries.[20] Another leading British publication, the *Edinburgh Medical Journal,* which continued until the mid-twentieth century, offers another suggestive comparison, for it was represented in major sets in only 34 libraries in the United States.

The citation profile of the BMJ

The evidence is clear that from the beginning, then, the *British Medical Journal* had significant presence in the United States and substantial interchange with American physicians. But it is still possible to go on and ask whether or not American medical personnel actually read the *BMJ.* Based on what happened in America, was the existence of the journal in world medicine more than ceremonial? It was to answer those questions that I undertook sampling the number of times material from the *BMJ* was actually cited in non-speciality American medical journals.[21]

Moreover, it is true that a journal, like any other institution, changes over time and can wax and wane as immediate circumstances and personnel and aspirations change. Only two general medical journals have lasted throughout the past 150 years in the United States, the *New England Journal of Medicine* and the *American Journal of the Medical Sciences.* In the cases of the *New England Journal,* the format of the journal only permits a tabulation that begins in the last part of the nineteenth century, but a very rough calculation, using *The Lancet* and to some extent the *Journal of the American Medical Association* for comparison, shows the proportion of citations that came from the

Table 9.1 Proportion of citations from the *BMJ*, compared with *The Lancet* and *JAMA*, in the *New England Journal of Medicine*

1891	7.6% (*Lancet* 7.9%; *JAMA* 2.3%)
1901	4.3%
1911	3.6% (*Lancet* 6.8%)
1921	2.8% (*Lancet* 2.4%; *JAMA* 2.6%)
1931	1.7% (*Lancet* 1.9%)
1941	1.2% (*Lancet* 2.2%; *JAMA* 9.3%)
1951	1.1% (*Lancet* 1.7%)
1961	2.3% (*Lancet* 4.0%; *JAMA* 4.9%)
1971	1.6% (*Lancet* 3.8%)
1981	1.7% (*Lancet* 5.3%; *JAMA* 1.8%)

BMJ in Table 9.1.

These raw figures and the comparisons that I have included require some comment. The two leading British journals, and the *BMJ* in particular, declined in the percentage of the citations in the *New England Journal* in the twentieth century. But after the Second World War, so did *JAMA*, which had become better cited by the middle of the twentieth century. It is certainly a fair inference from what is known about the explosion in biomedical publication that the competition in the second half of the twentieth century was extraordinarily keen. Moreover, the explosion took place particularly in the more scientific as opposed to the clinical areas, so that journals such as *BMJ* and *JAMA*, with strong clinical components (not to mention obligations to the sponsoring organizations), would naturally be at a disadvantage in the academicized world of biomedicine. The *BMJ* nevertheless maintained in the *New England Journal of Medicine* a consistent and respectable place among journals cited over a very long time, having reached some sort of low point around the time of the Second World War.

This profile in an American journal is strikingly parallel to the profile of the incidence of significant papers published in the *BMJ* as described by Bartrip.[22] The parallel between Bartrip's finding of significant papers and my profile citation certainly suggests that American citations do measure importance in the world of medicine in general.

Finally, and perhaps most important, what this one sample underlines – and I should state right off that a similar pattern appears in my other samples – is that the *BMJ* showed great lasting power. Why that was so is perhaps the most interesting question of all.

The *New England Journal of Medicine* was for some time a very parochial publication, tied closely to the local Boston medical community and sometimes the Harvard medical school. A check on the generality of trends among traditionally Anglophile Bostonians may perhaps be offered by another general journal with a different local base, the *New York State Journal of Medicine*, for which there is a full twentieth-century series, albeit within a context of variable quality as a journal (see Table 9.2). Especially in the early years, this sample is based on relatively small numbers (a total of only 240 references for 1916, for example, in contrast to 1101 for 1986). Yet the general patterns visible in the *New England Journal of Medicine* persist.

Table 9.2 Proportion of citations from the *BMJ*, compared with *The Lancet*, in the *New York State Journal of Medicine*

1906	3.1% (*Lancet* 7.3%)
1916	1.3% (*Lancet* 3.0%)
1926	4.1% (*Lancet* 1.9%)
1936	1.3% (*Lancet* 1.8%)
1946	3.2% (*Lancet* 1.1%)
1956	1.2% (*Lancet* 1.2%)
1966	1.4% (*Lancet* 1.2%)
1976	1.8% (*Lancet* 4.0%)
1986	0.9% (*Lancet* 2.8%)

There are also figures for the proportions of citations of the *BMJ* in the American medical journal that was patterned deliberately after the *British Medical Journal*, namely, the *Journal of the American Medical Association*, or *JAMA*, founded in 1883 (see Table 9.3).

As these figures confirm, it was clear, in the late nineteenth century, that *BMJ* and *Lancet* together cast a long shadow over the medical literature of the United States. But even later, in the *JAMA* samples as well as the others, the *BMJ* held throughout the twentieth century a very respectable place with, again, perhaps a little dip between the two world wars. And what the comparisons with other journals show is that two journals that I used in my sampling, namely, *The Lancet* and the *New England Journal of Medicine*, showed a remarkable relative rise, so that the comparisons are more of a comment on them than on the *BMJ*,

Table 9.3 Proportion of citations from the *BMJ*, compared with *The Lancet* and *NEJM*, in the *JAMA*

1883	12.2% (*Lancet* 9.8%)
1893	1.7% (*Lancet* 16.8%; *NEJM* 2.7%)
1903	6.9% (*Lancet* 5.0%; *NEJM* 2.4%)
1913	1.7% (*Lancet* 2.0%; *NEJM* 1.1%)
1923	1.4% (*Lancet* 2.2%; *NEJM* 0.04%)
1933	1.4% (*Lancet* 2.1%; *NEJM* 0.9%)
1943	1.5% (*Lancet* 2.9%; *NEJM* 1.1%)
1953	1.8% (*Lancet* 1.6%; *NEJM* 4.2%)
1963	2.2% (*Lancet* 3.3%; *NEJM* 2.8%)
1973	2.0% (*Lancet* 4.3%; *NEJM* 6.1%)
1983	1.4% (*Lancet* 4.7%; *NEJM* 7.4%)

which was relatively constant after the decline of all British journals, including *The Lancet*, just at the beginning of the century. The pattern for *JAMA* in the *New England Journal of Medicine*, by contrast, is much more variable, but it does confirm that the hierarchy apparent in data in the *Science Citation Index* in recent years existed for decades earlier.

Finally, all these conclusions can be tested by using samples from the oldest journal, the *American Journal of the Medical Sciences*, which was founded in 1820. In this case, from the beginning there were some references as well as abstracts, and I

Table 9.4 Proportion of citations from the *BMJ*, compared with *The Lancet*, in the *American Journal of the Medical Sciences*

1848	1%; abstracts 9.6% (*Lancet* 14.6% and 14.6%)
1858	2.3%; abstracts 5.7% (*Lancet* 9.5% and 6.9%)
1868	23.4% (*Lancet* 4.7%); combined figures
1878	10.8% (*Lancet* 14.2%); combined figures
1888	3.6%; abstracts 5.3% (*Lancet* 3.6% and 7.0%)
1898	11.9%; abstracts 6.2% (*Lancet* 4.0% and 1.6%)
1908	1.1%; abstracts 1.4% (*Lancet* 3.1% and 4.2%; *JAMA* 5.6% and 4.7%)
1918	2.6%; abstracts 7.0% (*Lancet* 2.4% and 3.9%)
1928	0.7%; abstracts 0.6% (*Lancet* 1.6% and 1.1%)
1938	3.0% (*Lancet* 6.4%)
1948	1.6% (*Lancet* 2.8%)
1958	1.2% (*Lancet* 1.7%)
1968	0.7% (*Lancet* 4.7%)
1978	2.4% (*Lancet* 3.7%; *JAMA* 2.7%)
1988	1.0% (*Lancet* 2.0%)

counted both (see Table 9.4).

The *American Journal of the Medical Sciences* in particular illustrates a number of problems with using citations to infer the history of journals. The variations in the figures often reflect accident and editorial policy. In fact, while the name remained the same, the *American Journal of the Medical Sciences* changed from a journal that was primarily a translator of foreign innovations in medical science for an American medical audience to a general medical journal and ultimately, in the late twentieth century, to a journal reflecting somewhat restricted research interests. Not only the *BMJ* but *The Lancet* and the *JAMA* appeared in it in a highly variable way.[23]

The persistence of the BMJ

In spite of complications, the figures from all the sample journals show the same steady decline in the twentieth century, as the *BMJ* and other journals had to compete with an enormous number of more or less highly specialized publications. In recent decades, for example, certain specialized journals in endocrinology would have surpassed all the general journals that I have tried to use for comparisons.[24] And the same would have been true, even in various general journals, at an earlier period when surgery was very central to medicine and the surgical journals were frequently cited.

One indication of the factor of competition is the changing proportion of citations to the various British biomedical journals. In the early years of the *BMJ* journals, the total for them combined with *The Lancet* was only a fraction of the total citations in the *American Journal of the Medical Sciences* taken from all British journals. By the late nineteenth century, the *British Medical Journal* and *The Lancet* had both risen in prestige so that references to them were a very large part of the British representation; in 1878 and 1898 they actually constituted a majority and represented a presence that raises that unanswerable question of how much, for many decades afterwards, both *BMJ* and *The Lancet* were cited simply because it was traditional to do so.

All these compiled numbers from leading American journals serve only to confirm the reality of impressions that will come to anyone who looks over a large number of medical journals from throughout the world. The figures nevertheless do indicate the gross magnitudes within which journals can be compared – magnitudes that changed from at least the late nineteenth century to the late twentieth century. From them all, the conclusion continues to obtrude: the *BMJ* persisted, even in a changing context.

Additional factors shaping citation data

One factor that biased the changing incidence of *BMJ* citations was the place of British medicine in the world. That the place of American medicine increased I have noted; but the course of medicine in Britain relative to the rest of the world was also not constant, although of course varying by specialty so that, at the turn of the century, UK work in, for example, parts of surgery was notable but in psychiatry backward, to say the least. Many historians have chronicled the problems of British medicine in the early and mid-nineteenth century, as opposed to achievements during the last decades of that century, and the citations also in fact confirm a general impression that British medicine played a larger part in world medicine after the Second World War than in earlier decades.[25]

Moreover, the nature of the medical article changed, from typically a paper reporting a personal experience or setting out a theoretical opinion, as in the middle of the nineteenth century, to a research report that by the late twentieth century often included hundreds of references that sometimes took up almost half the article. Such citation strategies represented adaptations to a world in which medical publications had multiplied so extraordinarily. L.E. Böttiger has recently suggested, as have others, that a large proportion of the citations in such lists were unnecessary and represented simply another form of practising defensive medicine.[26]

Still another complication, of course, was the fact that although a journal might have been published in a particular place, even under the aegis of a national medical organization, nevertheless the authors might work anywhere or be migrants. I have simply assumed (and I think not naively) that the incidence of such complications would be small enough that cross-national publishing (or, in the early days, pirating) would cancel out as a factor. But in so far as in the late twentieth century the biomedical world became truly international and also simultaneously anglophone, some of the problems of transmission that I have been raising became moot.

Penetrating the boundaries of national medical cultures

The reality for most of the past 150 years has been largely otherwise. There were national communities and even regional and local medical communities. At most there existed concurrently what Böttiger characterizes as 'an iron curtain surrounding the English-speaking' medical writers, who formed a community through mutual citation.[27] In fact, as my evidence suggests, even the movement of knowledge and practice from Britain to the United States had to breach formidable social, if not intellectual, boundaries.

Students of the cross-cultural movement of medical thinking have identified various ways in which medicine has been communicated. For the United States, perhaps the most dramatic demonstration was Thomas N. Bonner's, who showed that fifteen thousand physicians from the United States actually travelled to German-speaking countries from 1870 to 1914 to study medicine, usually at the University of Vienna. Moreover, it is notorious that surgeons, especially, travelled to learn and improve technique by personal observation. Russell C. Maulitz, too, has examined the transit of ideas by way of students, in this case very precisely the path that pathological anatomy took from France to Britain in the early nineteenth century. Indeed, he spells out that the movement of knowledge and practice

> was thus not simply a matter of knowledge flowing through the funnel of a text tradition. Nor was it simply a question of 'technology transfer' by which the stethoscope was taken to England. The process was rather one in which *experience*, from the dissection table and the hospital wards, flowed through the careers of multitudinous young Englishmen as they made the journey out and back.[28]

The significance of the BMJ as an institution

Is the journal, then, beside the point as a carrier from one culture to another? It may be, as students of scientific communication argue, that the journal article is an after-the-fact record or register for science. But the evidence also shows that the article has a vital place in the whole process by which scientific knowledge and practice are communicated and even communicated internationally.[29] In either case, recorder or carrier or both, it is clear that the *British Medical Journal* was a force in Anglo–American and presumably world medicine from the very beginning, when there was not much competition, and persisted remarkably right into the era of the proliferation of speciality publications.

It is in this way that patterns of citation lead to consideration of the nature of the *BMJ* as an institution, the prominence and steady endurance of which together constitute an important historical phenomenon.[30] It was not certain that the journal would persist as it did. The *Medical Times and Gazette* (1839–85), for example, was for years more conspicuously cited in American journals than was the *British Medical Journal* or *The Lancet*. But the *Medical Times and Gazette* did not last so that we could celebrate a 150th anniversary in 1989. Other British journals, too, failed, and Americans noticed, and paid attention to, the survivors.[31]

Why did the *BMJ* outlast most other journals? Sociologists would answer in institutional terms and observe that one reason for the healthy survival of the *BMJ* was that it embodied the interests of an important group, the British Medical Association. But in representing that group, the *BMJ* also embodied values and norms beyond the profession, that is, the values and norms of medicine in general. Why else would American – or any other – medical personnel cite the journal so often? As John Ziman emphasizes, a journal functions to show and enforce the cooperative solidarity of science and, we can add, the medical endeavour in general. The record of citations in fact is a very good measure of the effective institutional functioning – the impact – of a journal.[32]

It is in this light that the ability of the successive editors of the *BMJ* to maintain a significant presence in American medicine – furnishing at the least one or two out of every hundred citations over 150 years – is so impressive. Many writers have discussed both the editors of the *BMJ* and the editors of other journals, but such discussions tend to be general; precisely what medical editors over the centuries have done that is right or wrong remains extremely obscure, although Bartrip makes the case that one important element is the independence and critical abilities of an editor.[33]

By taking as a point of departure the success of the *BMJ* as an institution, we can get some perspective on the question of why it was so by taking from the sociologists a measure of how an institution makes an impact on society, in this case medicine. Repeatedly the editors of the *BMJ* led in shaping and setting norms, not just in the UK but in the world in general, and to maintain their place they had to adapt to and manipulate changes in British medicine, in American medicine, in the larger anglophone medicine, and in world medicine. The early and continuing interest of the editors in quality and expertise was reflected in the citations. So, too, was their sensitivity to both science and clinical application simultaneously. As John Maddox has observed, publication policies of journals influence the way in which scientists do experiments (for example, including control studies), and others have noted that communication shapes activities that are to be communicated.[34] A major element in the success of the *BMJ* lay not in the fact that the history of the journal embodied so much of the history of medicine, but that it embodied aspirations of the members of the profession in a way that transcended national cultures over a long period of time.

Notes

1. I have drawn freely from James Eckman, 'Anglo-American hostility in American medical literature of the nineteenth century', *Bulletin of the History of Medicine*, 1941, 9: 31–71. 'American estimate of native medical literature', *Provincial Medical and Surgical Journal*, 1849, 13: 196. See in general James H. Cassedy, 'The flourishing and character of early American medical journalism, 1797–1860', *Journal of the History of Medicine and Allied Sciences*, 1983, 38: 135–50; Genevieve Miller, 'The nineteenth century medical press', in John B. Blake (ed.), *Centenary of Index Medicus*, US Department of Health and Human Services, Public Health Service, National Library of Medicine (NIH Publication No. 80-2068), Bethesda, MD, 1980, pp. 19–29.

2. Eckman, 'Anglo-American hostility'; the quotation is from p. 46. 'Medical journals in America', *British Medical Journal*, 1883, 1: 68.

3. Eckman, 'Anglo-American hostility'. J. Greig Smith, 'Modern medical journalism', *Bristol Medico-Chirurgical Journal*, 1893, 11: 221.

4. The counts recorded in this paper are approximate only and usually cover only half or a quarter of each sample year. Book citations were not included. See further comments below.

5. Ramon Velez and Donald I. Patrick, 'Citation of foreign literature in U.S. and U.K. journals', *New England Journal of Medicine*, 1982, 307: 1155. Cf. Cl. Olivier, P. Casseyre and M. Vayssairat, 'Future of French-language journals', *Lancet*, 1989, 2: 222. L.E. Böttiger, 'Reference lists in medical journals – language and length', *Acta Medica*

Scandinavia, 1983, 214: 73–7, found 91% of the references in his international sample to be in English, while a sample Medline search showed only 59% of the world medical literature to be in English.

6. As Maurice Crosland has pointed out, any discussion of national science implicitly involves comparisons. But in talking about intercultural penetration, I am not talking about the question of national styles in science. Maurice Crosland, 'History of science in a national context', *British Journal for the History of Science*, 1977, 10: 95–113. Cf. John Theodore Merz, *A History of European Thought in the Nineteenth Century*, Edinburgh: William Blackwood and Sons, 1904, I, pp. 15–16 and *passim*; and Nathan Reingold, 'National style in the sciences: the United States case', in E.G. Forbes (ed.), *Human Implications of Scientific Advance; Proceedings of the XVth International Congress of the History of Science, Edinburgh 10–15 August 1977*, Edinburgh: Edinburgh University Press, 1978, pp. 163–73. Examples include Gerald L. Geison, *Michael Foster and the Cambridge School of Physiology; the Scientific Enterprise in late Victorian Society*, Princeton: Princeton University Press, 1978; Jonathan Harwood, 'National styles in science: genetics in Germany and the United States between the World Wars', *Isis*, 1987, 78: 390–414; cf. John C. Burnham, 'Instinct theory and the German reaction to Weismannism', *Journal of the History of Biology*, 1972, 5: 321–6. Nor am I talking about emphases on different specialties in different countries, which can also be measured by citation counts. A comparison by specialty is C. Zimmerman and P.A.J.M. Verhaak, *Het practisch tijdschrift voor de geneeskunde in al haren omvang, 1822–1856*, Nijmegen: KU Nijmegan Instituut voor Geschiedenis der Geneeskunde, Scripta Tironum no. 20, 1990, pp. 31–3.

7. J.M. Ziman, *Public Knowledge; an Essay concerning the Social Dimension of Science*, Cambridge: Cambridge University Press, 1968 especially pp. 102–6.

8. An excellent summary is Leonard Karel, 'Selection of journals for *Index Medicus*: a historical review', *Bulletin of the Medical Library Association*, 1967, 55: 259–78.

9. See, for example, the summary in William Goffman, 'Literature selection', in K.S. Warren (ed.), *Selectivity in Information Systems*, New York: Praeger, 1985, pp. 121–6; as well as Karel, 'Selection of journals'. A.J. Meadows, *Communication in Science*, London: Butterworths, 1974, chap. 6. The pioneer work based on citations was P.L.K. Gross and E.M. Gross, 'College libraries and chemical education', *Science*, 1927, 66: 385–9. See especially William Dosite Postell, 'Further comments on the mathematical analysis of evaluating scientific journals', *Bulletin of the Medical Library Association*, 1946, 34: 107–9.

10. N.S. Stearns and W.W. Ratcliff, 'An integrated health science care library for physicians, nurses, and allied health practitioners in community hospitals', *New England Journal of Medicine*, 1970, 283: 1490–7; R. Allyn, 'A library for internists III: recommended by the American College of Physicians', *Annals of Internal Medicine*, 1979, 90: 450–77; Jennie Gregory, 'An evaluation of medical periodicals', *Bulletin of the Medical Library Association*, 1937, 25: 172–88; Alfred N. Brandon, 'Selected list of books and journals for the small medical

library', *Bulletin of the Medical Library Association*, 1965, 53: 329–64; Alfred N. Brandon, Dorothy R. Hill and Gustave and Janet W. Levy, 'Selected list of books and journals for the small medical library', *Bulletin of the Medical Library Association*, 1989, 77: 139–69. Library of the American Medical Association, *Recent Books and Periodicals selected for the Small Medical Library*, Chicago: American Medical Association, 1959, p. 20. See, for example, Goffman, 'Literature selection', p. 125. There were many other studies reported over the years in the *Bulletin of the Medical Library Association*.

11. E. Garfield, 'Citation indexing for studying science', *Nature*, 1970, 227: 669–71. Derek Price early saw that in this new world of citation studies, in which importance could be measured quantitatively, every editor would aspire to issue the legendary *Journal of Really Important Papers*; Derek J. de Solla Price, 'Networks of scientific papers', *Science*, 1965, 149: 510–15. Eugene Garfield, 'Citation analysis as a tool in journal evaluating', *Science*, 1972, 178: 471–9. Eugene Garfield, 'Which medical journals have the greatest impact?' *Annals of Internal Medicine*, 1986, 105: 313–20. P.W.J. Bartrip, *Mirror of Medicine; A History of the British Medical Journal*, Oxford: British Medical Journal and Clarendon Press, 1990, p. 70–1. Cf. Eugene Garfield, *Ghostwriting and other Essays*, Philadelphia: ISI Press, 1986, p. 201, on surgical journals alone. In the last half of the century, the only area in which the *BMJ* was not consistently at the very top among medical journals was in the 'impact' factor, and even then the *BMJ* was still ahead of the pack. (The 'impact' simply meant the number of times each paper in the journal was cited in a given year, and it was meant to control the fact that, by publishing a large number of pages, such journals as *Lancet* and *JAMA* and *BMJ* contained more articles and so had an advantage in comparisons based solely on counting total citations; indeed, from the 1880s, the *BMJ* carried boasts of having a larger circulation and publishing more pages per year than any other medical journal.) But I should point out that this supposed quality factor of individual articles (which could also be a fad factor), the measurement of which is designed to equalize quarterlies and weeklies, is quite different from the question that I am raising, namely, the gross impact of an institution, in which the question is not the impact rate for individual articles but the total difference made over a long time by the existence of the journal.

12. Ernest Hart, 'Medical journalism', *Medical News*, 1893, 62: 655. Frank Luther Mott, *A History of American Magazines, 1885–1905*, Cambridge, MA: Harvard University Press, 1957, p. 529–30. Bartrip, *Mirror of Medicine*, p. 306.

13. See, for example, John T. Bruer, William Goffman and Kenneth S. Warren, 'Selective medical libraries and library networks for developing countries', *American Journal of Tropical Medicine and Hygiene*, 1981, 30: 1133–40.

14. David Walsh, 'On certain aspects of medical journalism', *Medical Press and Circular*, 1909, 88: 89. 'The journal's centenary', *British Medical Journal*, 1940, 2: 454. In 1857 there were 2,100 subscribers to the *British Medical Journal*; *British Medical Journal*, April 18, 1857, p. 325;

by 1900, there were more than 21,000 copies circulated and by 1924 more than 31,000. See Bartrip, *Mirror of medicine*, pp. 185, 217.

15. The total *BMJ* circulation for 1960 was about 83,000 and for 1989 about 104,000. I am greatly indebted to Mr Maurice Long for *BMJ* circulation figures, Other total circulation figures appear in Bartrip, *Mirror of Medicine*, p. 303. Circulation figures for American serials are in *Ayers*.

16. Roy M. Macleod, 'Securing the Foundations', *Nature*, 1969: 443–4. Bartrip, *Mirror of Medicine*, pp. 302–3, points out that both Hart and Clegg aspired to international eminence for the *BMJ*.

17. Meadows, *Communication in Science*, London: Butterworths, 1974, chap. 3. A.J. Meadows, 'Access to the results of scientific research: developments in Victorian Britain', in *idem.* (ed.), *Development of Science Publishing in Europe*, Amsterdam: Elsevier Science Publishers, 1980, pp. 50–3, comments on the rise of abstracting in science, which took a somewhat different turn from the traditional 'Periscope' abstracts sections of American medical journals. See also May F. Katzen, 'The changing appearance of research journals in science and technology: an analysis and a case study', in ibid., p. 207. (In the last half of the nineteenth century, it is true, a single journal was often assigned to one abstracter, who could be paid for the job. I would contend that, in the crude counting that I have done, these corrupting institutional influences were swamped over time by the simple persistence of importance.)

18. M. Roux, 'On resection of the elbow-joint', *Provincial Medical and Surgical Journal*, April 24, 1841: 70–1, reprinted in *American Journal of the Medical Sciences*, 1841, ns2: 201.

19. G.C.S., review of Bennett, *Clinical lectures on the principles and practice of medicine*, in *American Journal of the Medical Sciences*, 1858, 36: 431. R.H. Page, 'Relations of medical journalism to medical progress', *Country Practitioner*, 1879, 1: 5–8.

20. Frank Luther Mott, *A History of American Magazines, 1865–1885*, Cambridge, MA: Harvard University Press, 1938, p. 140. I would have liked to compare *The Lancet*, but it does not offer a proper comparison since from 1842 to 1892 the journal was reprinted in the United States.

21. The nature of the enquiry does not require a complex research protocol such as that suggested in Eugene Garfield, Irving H. Sher and Richard J. Torpie, *The Use of Citation Data in Writing the History of Science*, Philadelphia: Institute for Scientific Information, Inc., 1964. Likewise, for a first research, it is not necessary to accommodate to comments such as those of Böttiger that many citations are merely ceremonial.

22. Bartrip, *Mirror of Medicine*, pp. 121–5, 182.

23. A comparison of this variability is offered by a year-by-year tally of *BMJ* and *Lancet* in another leading American journal, the *Medical News*, from 1857 to 1893. Again, there were wide variations from year to year; only the general tendencies were clear:

1857–1858	10.0%	
1859–1861	11.9%	
1862	8.9%	(*Lancet* 23.2%)
1863	27.0%	

1864–1865	24.8%
1866–1867	28.6%
1868–1869	25.0%
1870–1871	26.9% (*Lancet* 20.2%)
1872–1873	40.5% (*Lancet* 37.3%)
1874–1875	12.5% (*Lancet* 35.8%)
1876–1877	17.1% (*Lancet* 30.8%)
1878–1879	39.3% (*Lancet* 16.1%)
1881	13.0% (*Lancet* 17.3%)
1882	11.3% (*Lancet* 15.9%)
1883	7.7% (*Lancet* 6.9%)
1884	7.2% (*Lancet* 9.2%)
1885	11.3% (*Lancet* 8.5%)
1886	10.8% (*Lancet* 15.3%)
1887	9.2% (*Lancet* 10.9%)
1888	13.4% (*Lancet* 9.8%)
1889	12.2% (*Lancet* 12.7%)
1890	8.7% (*Lancet* 8.0%)
1891	0.9% (*Lancet* 4.2%)
1892	11.3% (*Lancet* 7.5%)
1893	9.5% (*Lancet* 4.8%)

Other samples from the nineteenth century provide no further light and only confirm trends and changes already noted. And lest anyone be tempted to take my samplings too much at face value, let me indicate that in the early years, especially, the numerical basis of the sample is often very small and can account for wide swings that did not depend on editorial whim. In 1858 in the *American Journal of the Medical Sciences*, for example, there were in the whole year only 42 references/citations that could be counted (there were 261 abstracts), while in later years the samples ran to 1,000 or 2,000 before I stopped.

24. This was happening as early as the 1930s, according to Jennie Gregory, 'Evaluation of medical periodicals', *Bulletin of the Medical Library Association*, 1939, 27: 244. See, for example, John A. Timour, 'Selected lists of journals for the small medical library: a comparative analysis', *Bulletin of the Medical Library Association*, 1971, 59: 87–93; Gary D. Byrd and Michael E.D. Koenig, 'Systematic serials selection analysis in a small academic health sciences library', *Bulletin of the Medical Library Association*, 1978, 66: 397–406.

25. An interesting example using *Lancet* citations in a different medical culture is Annemarie van Eekelen, *Naar een rationele zuigelingen-voeding; voedingleer en kindergeneeskunde in Nederland (1840–1914)*, Nijmegen: Koninklijke drukkerij G.J. Thieme, 1984, pp. 95–6.

26. Böttiger, 'Reference lists in medical journals'. My sampling covered only journal articles, not books, although it is my impression that the results would not have differed materially. The *BMJ* did begin at a time when in American medical literature, at least, references in papers, if references were included at all, were to standard volumes and standard authors, not to 'medical newspapers'. By the late twentieth century, the references consisted almost entirely of journal articles rather than books, which surprisingly means the exclusion of

papers in edited books and symposia (a fact leading many biomedical scientists to publish redundantly in an indexed journal versions of material concurrently appearing in collected volumes). Since I was not prepared for the extent to which books disappeared from the literature, I did not do a formal count, but such a count would call into question the need for books in the medical field during most of the twentieth century. Böttiger also notes the minor place of books. Cf. Meadows, *Communication in Science*, p. 90.

27. Böttiger, 'Reference lists in medical journals', p. 77.

28. Thomas Neville Bonner, *American Doctors and German Universities; a chapter in international intellectual relations*, Lincoln: University of Nebraska Press, 1963. Russell C. Maulitz, *Morbid Appearances: the Anatomy of Pathology in the Early Nineteenth Century*, Cambridge: Cambridge University Press, 1987, especially p. 136.

29. Ziman, *Public knowledge*, chap. 6.

30. J.M. Ziman, 'Information, communication, knowledge', *Nature*, 1969, 224: 318.

31. Cassedy, *Early American Journalism*, p. 146.

32. See, for example, Robin M. Williams, Jr, 'Recent developments in research on social institutions', *Annals of the American Academy of Political and Social Science*, 1967, 374: 171–85. Ziman, *Public Knowledge*, chap. 6. See also Meadows, *Scientific communication*, pp. 172–4.

33. Bartrip, *Mirror of Medicine*, *passim* but especially pp. 314–15. A centenary evaluation of the parallel case of *Nature* was 'that *Nature* survived its first years by sheer journalism . . . honest . . . concern for the mutual interests of contributors and readers . . .'; 'Is it safe to look back?' *Nature*, 1969, 224: 419.

34. John Maddox, 'Can journals influence science?' *Nature*, 1989, 339: 657.

10

Psychiatric journals and the evolution of psychological medicine

Michael Shepherd

I have been asked to 'look generally at the development of psychiatric journals against the backdrop of psychiatric knowledge and the emerging specialism'. This is no easy task. The proliferation of medical journals in the nineteenth century was nowhere greater than in the field of psychiatry and, as Helen Marshall has pointed out:

> the general psychiatric journals reflect the history and nature of the subject. Their changes in title, like those of their parent societies, indicate changing concepts of and attitudes towards mental illness . . . Some of its [psychiatry] branches are esoteric, semantically confusing and often subtle, as journal titles sometimes show.[22]

Within the framework of this symposium the content as well as the titles of psychiatric journals may be viewed as markers of developments in theory and opinion as well as providers of factual information and I shall treat them as such, taking my examples from the British, American, German and French literature.

The journalistic mainstream arose in 1783 in Germany, with the publication of the significantly entitled *Gnothi Sauton, oder Magazin zur Erfahrungsseelenkunde für Gelehrte und Ungelehrte*, i.e. *Know Thyself, or a Magazine for Empirical Psychology for Scholars and Laymen*, to which was added *mit Unterstutzung mehrerer Wahrheitsfreunde*, i.e. *with the support of a number of friends of truth.*[13] The founding editor was Karl Philipp Moritz, a friend of Goethe and best-known for his novel, *Anton Reiser.* Moritz himself was anticlerical but not nihilistically so, as he demonstrated when his colleague, C.F. Pockels, attempted to steer the journal into a frankly atheistic posture. His primary concern was to wrest the study of human behaviour from the grasp of philosophy into the field of what we would now call the life sciences. In this aim he was in tune with his times. As one commentator has observed:

> the emergence of psychology in the Age of Enlightenment relates to the religious crisis of that time in this way: there is now a search for the certainties of religious life in individual experience rather than through conformity to a particular set of cosmological and theological views. The interest of that age in the 'a priori' categories of experiencing as developed by Kant can be seen both in relation to the religious crisis of that time and to the developing psychology.[12]

These extracts from the prospectus outlined in the first issue of Moritz's journal indicate what he had in mind:

> *Sketch of basic considerations with regard to a psychopathology*
>
> In a magazine of empirical psychology there should be as few inserted reflections as possible, particularly in the beginning. Later it can develop through the mutual assistance of significant reflections and facts.
>
> All anxious efforts to attain a closed system are to be avoided, and everything is to remain a tentative sketch, in which any line can once more be removed, even though as a whole it should thereby take on an altogether different form . . .
>
> 1. Lack of relative harmony of all psychic capacities is psychic illness (Seelenkrankheit).
>
> This depends not so much on the strength or weakness of a particular psychic capability and of itself, but rather on how far, with regard to the remaining psychic capabilities, it is either too strong or too weak . . .
>
> 2. These disturbances of the necessary proportion among the psychic capabilities often resolve themselves; only when they persist are they genuine illness . . .
>
> 3. Since psychic illnesses arise from various causes, there is certainly no panacea for them. The moral doctor must

> study these illnesses in terms of their manifestations, their causes and sequelae, if he wishes to try to cure them . . .
> 4. Are moral doctors possible, and have they existed? Socrates seems to have understood and practised this sublime art to the very highest degree.

The contributors to Moritz's journal included lawyers, teachers and clergymen as well as physicians, and their writings covered a broad spectrum of topics: case reports of abnormal or unusual behaviour, the structure of language, pedagogy, 'action without consciousness of motives, or the power of obscure ideas', and the relationship between psychology and religion. In 1792 the theologian David Mauchart produced the *Allgemeines Repertorium für empirische Psychologie und verwandte Wissenschaften (General Repertory of Empirical Psychology and Related Sciences)*, but by and large philosophers tended to be readier than theologians to associate themselves with these trends, as in Kant's famous booklet on mental hygiene, and in 1805 Johann Christian Reil founded the journal *Magazin für psychische Heilkunde* with the philosopher, Kayssler.[18] Reil also collaborated with another philosopher Johann Christian Hoffbauer, to produce the *Beiträge zur Beforderung einer Curmethode auf psychischem Wege (Contributions to the Advancement of Psychological Therapies)*, but not until 1818 did Friedrich Nasse, one of Reil's followers, bring out the *Zeitschrift für psychische Arzte (Journal for Psychological Doctors)*, the first German periodical under sole medical direction, and one which continued for five years.[25] While philosophers and theologians were involved in its production, the thrust of the journal was away from Romantic Naturphilosophie and towards the notion that the study of mental disease should be an integral part of medicine. In 1823, Nasse followed this journal with his *Zeitschrift für Anthropologie*, drawing on the contemporary philosophical ideas about human nature which constituted the 'anthropology' of the day.

Meanwhile, the first crop of mental hospitals was in the process of construction. In 1837 Nasse and Maximilian Jacobi produced the *Zeitschrift für die Beurteilung und Heilung der krankhaften Seelenzustände* explicitly for directors of psychiatric institutions, and 1844 saw the arrival of a national journal, the *Allgemeine Zeitschrift für Psychiatrie und psychische und gerichtliche Medizin (The General Journal for Psychiatry, Mental and Legal Medicine)*, which remained in existence for more than 100 years as the central vehicle of publication for the new profession of institutional psychiatry.

Within a brief period the alienists working in mental hospitals in other countries produced journals to serve the same purpose. In France the *Annales Médico-psychologique*, envisaged by Pinel decades earlier, had appeared one year previously, in 1843, following the passage of the Loi sur Les Aliénés in 1838.[8] The *Journal de Médecine Mentale* followed in 1861[10] and the *Annales de Psychiatrie* in 1891, when the word 'psychiatry' at last entered the French language. In the United States the *American Journal of Insanity*, the first psychiatric journal in the English language, was established in 1844 and, it has been observed, 'was undoubtedly a factor in the formation of the Association of Medical Superintendents of American Institutions for the Insane four months after the Journal was founded'.[3] The creation of the Association of American Institutions for the Insane, incidentally, led to a cleavage between hospital superintendents and the prison reformers, whose views were represented by the *Journal of Prison Discipline and Philanthropy*, founded in 1845. The confinement of many insane people in jails was resented by hospital doctors who wished to remove the stigma of criminality from lunacy. In Germany their acknowledgement of the legal implications of their medical practice, however, was indicated by the inclusion of 'legal medicine' in the title of the *Allgemeine Zeitschrift*. The concept of legal anthropology (gerichtliche Anthropologie) had been introduced by Johann Baptist Friedrich who developed a special interest in what was to become forensic psychiatry. Friedrich, it may be noted, was an early example of the emerging species of the committed medical journalist and was responsible for no fewer than four short-lived psychiatric journals with a forensic input in the early years of the nineteenth century – *Archiv für Psychologie für Arzte und Juristen* (1834), *Magazin für die philosophische medizinische und gerichtliche Seelenkunde* (1829–31), *Fortsetzung* (1832) and *Blättern für Psychiatrie* (1837–38). He also attempted unsuccessfully to bring out a *Bibliothek der deutschen Medizin und Chirurgie* in 1837 and, undaunted, as late as 1850 he produced *Blättern für gerichtliche Anthropologie*.

In Britain the official organ of the Association of Medical Officers of Asylums and Hospitals for the Insane was launched in 1855. This was named the *Asylum Journal*, later the *Asylum Journal of Mental Science*, so called because, in the words of the editor:

> Our journal does not contain a single article which can truly be called *psychological*. Its character is strictly *psychiatric*, and the matters discussed in its pages are restricted to such as have immediate reference to the pathology and therapeutics of insanity, to the construction and management of asylums, and to the diseases, accidents and difficulties likely to arise therein.[7]

Here was the credo of psychiatry conceived in terms of what Gerald Grob has called 'an administrative specialty'.[15] In 1853 the Report of the Commissioners in Lunacy defined the province of the medical superintendent of the public asylum. The consequences were profound, and led to what a modern medical historian has called the

> division of psychiatrists into two groups of specialists within the specialty, each with different experience of a different type and class of patient – and even with its own journal – which has persisted more or less to this day and left its mark not only on the practice but even on the theory of psychiatry. Consulting physicians disenfranchised from public asylum practice tended to concentrate on the earlier milder and socially superior cases in private practice, while the new group of asylum medical officers treated mainly the poor and severely disturbed. This practical division of psychiatrists into those without and those within asylums having little contact because faced with different problems, fostered a theoretical division of mental illness into milder forms of neuroses so-called and severer forms of psychoses – the former treated by individual attention to individual problems which later developed into psychotherapy.[17]

An early editorial in the first issue of the *Asylum Journal* indicates the extent of the split:

> It is the opinion of an eminent contemporary . . . that the 'posts of resident medical officers to our county lunatic asylums' are not sought for, and therefore are not occupied by the 'best and highest class of psychological physicians' . . . It is sufficiently intelligible why the London specialist should desire to find himself attached

> officially to some great asylum, and to gild the solid pudding of lucrative private practice with the honour of public distinction. But what time could a metropolitan 'psychological physician of the best and highest class' find in which to study the peculiarities of thought, habit, and disposition, of some hundreds, or say a thousand, of insane paupers? What leisure to obtain the smallest insight into their characters? What chance of gaining the slightest influence over them? We apprehend that even the overworked and underpaid resident may find greater opportunity for intellectual culture, than such a person with his private practice, and his private asylums, and his public societies, and his various other psychological devices for obtaining name, and fame, and money . . . There is but little analogy and much contrast between the asylum and the general hospital.[6]

This was the point, then, in Britain and elsewhere, at which the main stream of psychiatry began to divide, and the journals of the day reflect the dichotomy. The establishment of the asylum provided a focal point for the new class of medical superintendents and their colleagues and it is not, therefore, surprising to find the pages of their association journal dominated by topics of primarily institutional concern – administrative issues, infections, hospital statistics, and clinical descriptions of severe mental illness. Asylum doctors were understandably less interested in Forbes Winslow's *The Journal of Psychological Medicine and Mental Pathology* which had appeared in 1848 and took a much broader view of the medical approach to mental disorder. Winslow regarded the term 'psychology' as synonymous with 'all that relates to the soul or mind of man in contradistinction to his material nature' and he promoted the concept of the 'psychological physician' as opposed to and transcending that of the alienist.[32] In his concern to emphasize psychology and philosophical enquiry in relation to mental disorder he was focusing on those broad issues which had stimulated Moritz to found his journal 65 years earlier and was reflecting the impact of Ernst von Feuchtersleben's seminal book, *The Principles of Medical Pathology*, which had been published in 1844, and translated into English in 1847.[34] This course of lectures for medical students was designed for

> not only . . . the psychiatric practitioners in lunatic asylums but . . . physicians in general, everyone of whom ought to have a clear view of the relations of the body to the mind . . . an exposition of all the relations under which mental operations may be represented to medical observation and medical treatment.[34]

Unlike the alienists, however, the advocates of psychological medicine were fragmented, being subjected to the influence of two new and quite separate disciplines, namely psychology and neurology. Each demands separate consideration.

The impact of psychology derived from two very different sources. The first of these can be traced to the late eighteenth century via its role in the development of the mental healing movement, stemming from the important influence exercised by Franz Anton Mesmer whose work on animal magnetism opened the door to a preoccupation with hypnosis. Gravitz has compiled a list of more than 130 journals devoted exclusively to hypnosis as a specialty in the past 200 years, omitting journals carrying a high proportion of articles on the subject.[14] The largest group of these journals was published in French. The first of them to be devoted exclusively to hypnosis was the *Annales de la Société Harmonique des Amis-Réunis de Strasbourg*, published in 1786, and the links between medical hypnosis and psychopathology were forged by a long line of distinguished nineteenth-century workers, including not only physicians like Liébault, Bernheim, Charcot and Janet, but also psychologists like Ribot and Binet. The influence of Mesmer's ideas is indicated by the way in which Nasse added to the original title of his *Zeitschrift für psychische Arzte*, the qualifying subtitle *mit besonderer Berücksichtung des Magnetismus (Journal for Psychological Doctors with special reference to Magnetism)* in 1820. The first anglophonic journal devoted to mesmerism, the *Magnetiser's Magazine and Annals of Animal Magnetism*, was published in London in 1816. Not until 1842 did the first three American journals appear, and the subsequent nineteenth-century history of mental healing in the US was a stormy one, involving religious and philosophical cults as well as schools of medical thought, all with their corresponding journals.[27]

Mention should also be made of phrenological periodicals, such as *Transactions of the Phrenological Society* (1821) and *The Phrenological Journal* (1824). For much of the nineteenth century, however, the links between the mental healing movement and the emerging medical specialty of psychiatry was tenuous. The most influential figure in bringing it into the medical orbit was undoubtedly Sigmund Freud. Regardless of the scientific value of his contributions, Freud's 'lasting achievement', according to Hearnshaw, 'was to have brought psychologists face to face with the whole range of human problems',[16] and from the outset he and his colleagues were well aware of the importance of propagating their ideas via journals as well as books. Shortly after the First International Psychoanalytical Congress in 1908 the first volumes of the *Jahrbuch* appeared, to be followed by the *Zentralblatt* (1910), the *Zeitschrift* (1912), *Imago* (1912), the *Psychoanalytic Review* (1913), the *Rundbriefe* (1919) and the *International Journal of Psychoanalysis* (1920). Since the 1920s such journals have proliferated in many languages, and so-called dynamic psychology has permeated nominally more general journals. The *Journal of Medical Psychology* is a case in point. Founded as the Medical Section of the *British Journal of Psychology* in 1920, it assumed its present name three years later. While the editor of this journal has always been medically qualified, between 1937 and 1975 he was a psychoanalyst and the present editor, a member of the scientific staff of an MRC unit, has recently affirmed that the journal is 'most aligned with psychotherapy' which he regards as a virtually independent activity no longer closely linked with either medicine or psychoanalysis.[2]

In contrast to the psychology of mental healing, academic psychology did not arise until the later half of the nineteenth century. As late as 1877, for example, the Senate of the University of Cambridge turned down a proposal to introduce the study of experimental psychology on the grounds that it would 'insult religion by putting the human soul in a pair of scales'. By contrast, in Germany a more open-minded attitude had fostered the development of psychology as an academic discipline, the offspring of philosophical psychology and the newly developing life sciences, especially physiology, in the German universities of the mid-nineteenth century. The key figure in this development was Wilhelm Wundt (1832–1920) who in 1875 was appointed professor of philosophy at Leipzig where he established a Psychological Institute four years later. In 1881 he brought out his journal, *Philosophische Studien*, which continued until 1903 as an organ of the Leipzig laboratory.

The first anglophonic periodical to be devoted entirely to this form of scientific psychology was *The American Journal of Psychology*, founded by G. Stanley Hall in 1897. Hall was disarmingly frank about the birth of his journal, which arose from the visit of

> a wealthy stranger from Philadelphia, J. Pearsall Smith, who had heard of a new department of psychology and who suggested that I start a journal, handing me on the spot a cheque for five hundred dollars to that end, with the intimation that more would follow . . . That was the origin of the American Journal of Psychology.[9]

For Hall the objective of the journal was 'to record the psychological work of a scientific, as distinct from a speculative, character', and it was aimed at a variegated readership, including '. . . teachers of psychology in higher institutions of learning; biologists and physiologists; anthropologists who are interested in primitive manifestations of psychological laws; physicians who give special attention to nervous and mental diseases; all others interested . . . in applying more exact methods to the study of the problems of human feelings, will and thought'. The intention was to accept 'studies in abnormal psychology, including the insane, criminals, idiotic, blind, deaf or other defectives or degenerates . . . the anthropology of myth, custom, religious belief, symbols, etc. among savage and ethnic stocks . . . genetic psychology and exact and careful child-study by scientific observers . . . animal psychology . . . neurological researches' and 'the psychology of philosophy, ethics, aesthetics, theology, etc'.

Hall claimed that his journal was radically different from its progenitor, *Mind*, which had appeared in 1876 edited by Croom Robertson, professor of philosophy and logic at University College, London. *Mind* purported to be 'the first English journal devoted to psychology and philosophy' but also represented the view that psychology could never be linked with the natural sciences. Nevertheless, only 30 years later, in 1904, the *British Journal of Psychology* appeared with an editorial which claimed that 'Psychology which till recently was known among us chiefly as Mental Philosophy, and was mainly concerned with problems of a more or less speculative character, has now at length attained the position of a positive science'.

This was merely one of a number of psychological journals which emerged at the turn of the century to reflect the growing impact of the subject. In 1890 there appeared the German *Zeitschrift für Psychologie und Physiologie der Sinnesorgane*. In France *L'Année Psychologique* was founded in 1894 and the *Journal de Psychologie Normal et Pathologique* in 1901.[26] Spain produced the *Revista di Psicologia* in 1905. In the United States, the *Psychological Review* appeared in 1894, *Psychological Monographs* and the *Psychological Index* in 1895. And with the journals came the societies: the American Psychological Association in 1892, the British Psychological Society and the Société Française de Psychologie in 1901, and the Deutsche Gesellschaft für Psychologie in 1904.

The increase in personnel and in the products of the psychological industry has been phenomenal. In 1932 C.M. Louttit was able to list 1,084 journals in his *Handbook of Psychological Literature*, along with a host of other published material in several languages.[21] Reviewing the content of this huge output he observed:

> The literature of psychology, like that of many other sciences, is to be found in widely scattered journals. Psychological materials comprise a large portion of the journals of psychiatry, psychoanalysis, philosophy, child-study, physiology and neurology; many articles are to be found in periodicals of general science, biology, zoology, anthropology, genetics, medicine, etc.; while several of the better class of popular magazines carry not-too-popular articles on psychological subjects. The fact that papers appear in such widely separated media makes it impossible to be familiar with the whole literature.

Sixty years ago, therefore, the original theoretical and experimental fields of psychology were already overshadowed by its many applications which Louttit tabulated by both subject and country. Abnormal psychology, i.e. psychology applied to morbid states, figured prominently in the listed journals, impinging on psychiatry, psychoanalysis, neurology, phrenology and magnetism. Further, the number of national journals was significantly related to the number of workers in each country, and a chronological analysis showed the point in time when the

United States overtook Germany as the most productive country in the field, a trend which was rapidly emphasized with the decline of German science after 1933. In terms of numbers, the American presence is now dominant. For example, the size of the membership of the American Psychological Association (APA), founded in 1892, has increased from a few hundred to well over 70,000. In 1982 the number of divisions within the APA had risen to 42, many of them quasi-independent, and the published output has grown correspondingly. Thus *Psychological Abstracts,* established in 1927, contained in its first year 2,730 abstracts from 267 journals; 50 years later there were 27,003 from almost 700 journals.

In the post-war period the publishing industry has expanded greatly and new psychology journals, many of them short-lived, have proliferated. It is, indeed, no longer possible to provide an accurate estimate of their numbers. Here, for example, is a list of titles of new journals recently advertised by a single American publisher: *Phobia Practice and Research Journal, Journal of Near-Death Studies* (formerly *Anabiosis*), *International Journal of Comparative Psychology, Journal of Marketing for Mental Health, Journal of Gay and Lesbian Psychotherapy, Journal of Pastoral Psychotherapy, Journal of College Student Psychotherapy, Journal of Chemical Dependency Treatment, Drugs and Society, Journal of Psychology and Human Sexuality,* and *Loss, Grief and Care.*

One other point calls for comment. Though psychology as a discipline is much concerned with individuals, the growth of social psychology has extended its range in two other directions, namely the influence of other people on the behaviour of individuals, and the impact of cultural factors on the process of socialization. As such its links with both sociology and social anthropology have been close and all three disciplines have produced many journals of their own through which those aspects of their work impinging on mental abnormality have been published. Durkheim's work on suicide, to take one important example, would fall into this category and much of his work was published in *L'Année Sociologique* which he founded in 1895. Vice versa, Talcott Parsons, the eminent American sociologist who underwent psychoanalysis to try and understand its links with personality and social situations, published several key articles in the journal *Psychiatry.*

Apart altogether from psychology, however, the social dimensions of behaviour were to be more directly related to medicine, including psychiatry, through the empirical study of society that grew out of the statistical movement and found its expression in the social surveys and censuses which commenced in the nineteenth century and led to the emergence of public health as a medical concept. This ecological approach to human behaviour was clearly related to the notion of the epidemiology of disease and as public health workers came to include non-infectious as well as communicable diseases within their remit psychiatry began to figure increasingly in the subject-matter of journals devoted to mental health or mental hygiene rather than to mental illness. The activities of the mental health section of the American Public Health Association is representative of this trend which is reflected in the articles on mental health published in the *American Journal of Public Health* which was founded in 1911. Williams and Westermeyer have analysed these papers over the subsequent 75 years to show the fluctuations which they related to federal funding for mental health programmes.[31] The content of these articles is dominated by social issues, preventive measures and, above all, by epidemiological research and its application to mental health services.

The principal links between psychiatry and general medicine, however, were forged by the evolving specialty of neurology, once described by the late Lord Brain as 'the queen of medicine, which embraces in its scope the neurotropic virus and the human mind'. Each country developed its own pattern according to a host of local factors, and the complex relationship between the two disciplines is well expressed by the history of its journals.

In Germany the dominant influence of Wilhelm Griesinger led quickly to the development of an academic discipline of psychiatry within university medical schools conjoined with neurology.[1] His *Archiv für Psychiatrie und Neurologie*, founded in 1864, symbolized this trend which by the end of the century resulted in the establishment of a monolithic medical specialty based ultimately on the view of mental diseases as particular forms of cerebral disorder.

A completely different pattern developed in the US, where medicine was much less centralized and where university medicine had still to flower. The situation is reflected in the vagaries of the privately owned *Journal of Nervous and Mental Disease*, founded in 1874, which reflected the fissiparous tensions over three subsequent generations. The first issue contained this statement of editorial policy:

> The field we have especially in view is that of the nervous system, not only on it own account, but that of its relations to the body of which it forms a part, on the one hand, and to the mind and mental action on the other. It is not our intention to produce a Journal of Insanity. We leave this more restricted and important field to other journals. In our own country it is already occupied, with marked ability, by the American Journal of Insanity, now so well known, not alone to the profession in the United States but also in other lands. But we do not expect to neglect mental disease, clearly arising out of organic nervous disease.[4]

Under its first editor, J.S. Jewell, from 1874 to 1881, the journal published chiefly neurophysiological and neuropathological articles, but the editorials were much concerned with mental hospital reform and other forward-looking psychiatric issues and represented the views of the American Neurological Association in attacking those of the American Association of Asylum Superintendents, the forerunner of the American Psychiatric Association. Indeed, twenty years after the founding of the American Neurological Association in 1875 the *Journal of Nervous and Mental Disease* became its official organ in 1895. From 1882 to 1901 Jewell's various successors re-emphasized the emphasis on neurology and its related disciplines; the attitude towards psychiatry was to maintain concern for reform while decrying its low scientific standards.[5] Significantly, in 1892 two non-medical editors were appointed, one a neurophysiologist and the other an experimental psychologist whose function was to promote psychology as a basic science for psychiatry.

The next editor, Smith Ely Jelliffe, was at the helm from 1902 to 1944.[19] He brought psychiatry back into the foreground and from 1905 developed an increasing interest in psychotherapy and psychoanalysis. Editorial work was his occupational passion; in addition to the *Journal of Nervous and Mental Disease* he had a hand in editing *The Psychoanalytic Review, Medical News, The New York Medical Journal, The Transactions of the American Neurological Association, The Journal of Pharmacology* and the *Nervous and Mental Disease Monograph* series. He was succeeded by Nolan Lewis and J.D. Finesinger, and then by the current editor, E.B. Brody, who has emphasized the importance of the behavioural sciences for psychiatry. With the *Journal of Nervous and Mental Disease* moving towards psychiatry it was perhaps inevitable that the Board of Trustees of the American Medical Association should decide to establish a journal of their own to replace it as the official organ of the American Neurological Association.[20] In 1919 this duly appeared as the *Archives of Neurology and Psychiatry* but in 1957 there developed separate sections for each specialty, culminating two years later in the production of two journals, the *Archives of General Psychiatry* and the *Archives of Neurology*.

Britain was to present another variation on the same theme. The six volumes of the *Reports of the West Riding Asylum*, published between 1871 and 1876, were edited by the superintendent James Crichton-Browne, who attracted the interest of such eminent neurologists as David Ferrier and John Hughlings Jackson. The *Reports* preceded the appearance of the Journal *Brain* in 1878, edited originally by two psychiatrists (Crichton-Brown and John Bucknill) and two neurologists (Ferrier and Hughlings Jackson), but eight years later this was taken over by the Neurological Society of London and became increasingly an organ of clinical neurology and neurophysiology. This cannibalistic process was to prove the rule, as many neurologists began to make their reputations out of organic disease and their income out of mental disorder. Psychiatry, for them, as Adolf Meyer pointed out 50 years ago, was a 'mere subordinated appendix, useful for diplomatic reasons'.[23]

In 1902 there appeared the *Review of Neurology and Psychiatry*, in which the need for combining the two disciplines was explicitly stated in the first issue:

> 'The British Medical Schools,' said the author, 'are surely to be congratulated on the production of a journal in which the subjects of Neurology and Psychiatry are to be dealt with in combination. During the 19th century, and especially during the last 50 years, the students of scientific medicine, and also the practical clinician have recognised with steadily increasing conviction or the importance, the essential unity of the 2 subjects.'[30]

Unity here, however, was achieved by the domination of the neurologists whose interests were largely reflected in the balance of the published articles. In 1920 the *Review* was succeeded by the *Journal of Neurology and Psychopathology* which was then taken over by the British Medical Association in 1926 and renamed the *Journal of Neurology and Psychiatry*, but again with a neurologist as editor and relatively little psychiatric representation. This was nominally one of the three major British interwar journals of psychiatry, along with the *Journal of Mental Science* and the *LCC Archives of Neurology and Psychiatry*, which brought together the work of the Maudsley Hospital from the 1920s. In 1938 it was re-named the *Journal of Neurology and Psychiatry*, once more with a neurologist as editor and no more than a sprinkling of psychiatrists on the board. In 1948 it incorporated neurosurgery as a separate specialty to become the *Journal of Neurology, Neurosurgery and Psychiatry*. By the time I joined the editorial board in the early 1960s the proportion of psychiatric papers per annum was less than 1.0 per cent and after discussion with the editor of the *BMJ* I suggested, first, that the journal should cease to pay lip-service to psychiatry by severing its links with the subject and devoting itself solely to neurology and neurosurgery and, second, that the BMA create a new specialist journal devoted to psychological medicine in the original, larger sense of the term.

The proposal was warmly supported by the whole editorial board until it was pointed out that the great majority of subscribers to the journal were North American psychiatrists who would be unlikely to continue their subscriptions if the recommendation were adopted. At this point there was a sharp U-turn of opinion, with mutterings about tradition and the importance of preserving an image. The second proposal, however, was accepted and for a while the BMA continued to publish two ostensibly psychiatric journals until the position became clearly untenable. A glance at the *Journal of Neurology, Neurosurgery and Psychiatry* demonstrates that not much has changed since that time. Like the *Korsakow Journal of Neuropathology and Psychiatry* of the Soviet Union it remains dominated by articles focused on organic disease of the central nervous system. Elsewhere psychiatry and neurology have gone their separate ways, and journals like the *Archives of Neurology and Psychiatry* (1969), the *Acta Psychiatrica Scandinavica* (1961) and many of the French journals[24] have split into two separate publications.

In historical perspective, then, a bird's eye view of psychiatric journals facilitates an understanding of their complex development from several sources. The first of these originated with the gradual recognition, some 200 years ago, that the study of the mind belonged as much to medicine and psychology as to philosophy and theology. At approximately the same time a largely independent source can be traced to the emergence of the attempts to document and investigate the long-recognized phenomena associated with the psychotherapeutic aspects of magical and religious healing. In the mid-nineteenth century the unity of the first stream was split by the rise of professional psychiatric associations whose journals were focused principally on institutional matters. The extramural components of psychiatry became increasingly involved with the newer disciplines of neurology on the one hand, and psychology and other social sciences on the other, each with their appropriate journals. The twentieth century has witnessed a confluence of these various tributaries, the waters being reinforced and muddied by the metamorphosis of dynamic psychology in the form of psychoanalysis and its offshoots. An admixture of these many disciplines has now so inundated the field of psychiatry as to have given rise to material for an expanding number of diverse journals. The information scientists are well aware of the situation, which Elliott has illustrated diagrammatically[11] (see Figure 10.1).

It is apparent, therefore, that psychological medicine today embraces a federation of elements which have still to be effectively coordinated. In this regard, however, it does not differ from medicine as a whole. The philosopher, Gilbert Ryle, has defined medicine as no more than 'the name of a somewhat arbitrary consortium of more or less loosely connected inquiries and techniques'[28] and his brother, John Ryle, one of the most eminent physicians of the century, argued forcibly that these methods are not all somatic since 'more than half of practical medicine is psychology'.[29] From this perspective, psychological medicine is not so much a medical specialty as an extension of medicine itself, one to be practised by all who lay claim to the status of Moritz's 'moral doctor' or Winslow's 'psychological physician'.[33] Its journals tell a tale which the profession often prefers to ignore.

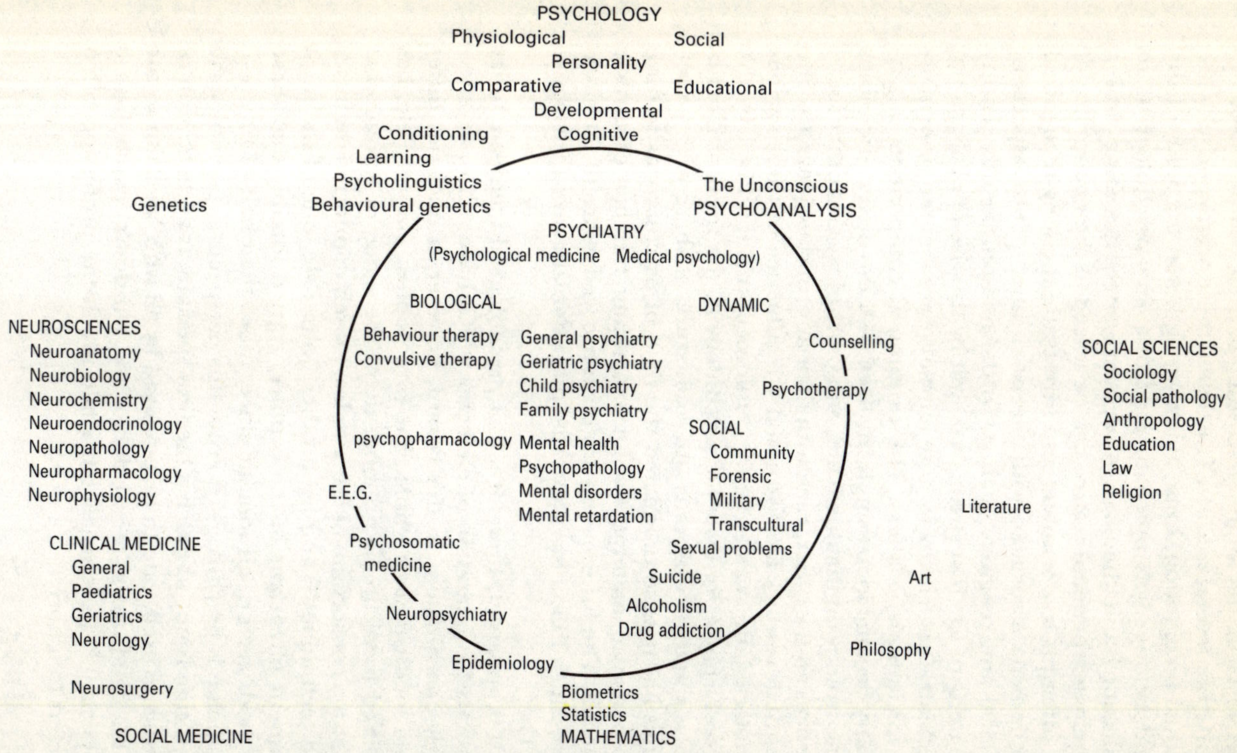

Figure 10.1 **Psychiatry and its related disciplines (Adapted from Elliott, 1971)**

Notes

1. E.H. Ackerknecht, *Kurze Geschichte der Psychiatrie*, Stuttgart: Enke Verlag, 1967.

2. J. Birtchnell, Editorial, *British Journal of Medical Psychology*, 1990, 63: 1–3.

3. F.J. Braceland, 'On editing the journal: Ave Atque Vale', *American Journal of Psychiatry*, 1978, 135: 1148–55.

4. E.B. Brody, 'The Journal of Nervous and Mental Disease: the first 100 years. I. 1874–1881', *The Journal of Nervous and Mental Disease*, 1974, 158: 6–17.

5. E.B. Brody, 'The Journal of Nervous and Mental Disease: the first 100 years. II. 1882–1901', *The Journal of Nervous and Mental Disease*, 1974, 159: 1–11.

6. J.C. Bucknill, 'Visiting Physicians to County Asylums', *The Asylum Journal*, 1854, 1, No. 3: 33–6.

7. J.C. Bucknill, Editorial, *Asylum Journal of Mental Science*, 1855, 2: 11.

8. R. Charpentier, 'Le centenaire des Annales Médico-psychologiques', *Annales Médico-psychologiques*, 1943, 101: 1–29.

9. K.M. Dallenbach, 'The American Journal of Psychology: 1887–1937', *The American Journal of Psychology*, 1937, 50: 489–506.

10. M. Delassiauve, 'Notre but', *Journal de Médecine Mentale*, 1861, 1: 1–4.

11. C.K. Elliott, *A Guide to the Documentation of Psychology*, Bingley, Linnet Books, 1971.

12. E. Eng, 'Karl Philipp Moritz's Magazin zur Erfahrungsseelenkunde (Magazine for Empirical Psychology) 1783–1793', *Journal of the History of the Behavioural Sciences*, 1973, 9: 300–5.

13. H. Förstl, M. Angermeyer and R. Howard, 'Karl Phillip Moritz's Journal of Empirical Psychology (1783–1793): an analysis of 124 case reports', *Psychological Medicine*, 1991, 21: 299–304.

14. M.A. Gravitz, 'Two Centuries of Hypnosis Specialty Journals', *The International Journal of Clinical and Experimental Hypnosis*, 1987, XXXV, No. 4: 265–76.

15. G.N. Grob, *Mental Institutions in America*, New York, The Free Press, 1973.

16. L. Hearnshaw, *The Shaping of Modern Psychology*, London: Routledge & Kegan Paul, 1987, pp. 156–7.

17. R. Hunter and I. MacAlpine, *Three Hundred Years of Psychiatry*, Oxford: Oxford University Press, 1963, pp. 1010–11.

18. G. Keil, 'Deutsche psychiatrische Zeitschriften des 19 Jahrhunderts', in G. Keil and G. Nissen (eds), *Psychiatrie auf dem Weg zur Wissenschaft*, Stuttgart: Thieme, 1985, pp. 28–35.

19. L.S. Kubie, 'The Journal of Nervous and Mental Disease: the first 100 years. III. 1902–1944', *The Journal of Nervous and Mental Disease*, 1974, 159, 77–80.

20. N.D.C. Lewis, 'The Journal of Nervous and Mental Disease: the first 100 years. IV. Century of service', *Journal of Nervous and Mental Disease*, 1974, 159, 319–23.

21. C.M. Louttit, *Handbook of Psychological Literature*, Bloomington, Indiana: The Principia Press, 1932.

22. H. Marshall, 'Psychiatry', in L.T. Morton (ed) *Use of Medical Literature*, London, Butterworth, 1975, pp. 306–32.

23. A. Meyer, 'The psychological point of view', in M. Bentley and M.V. Cowdrey (eds) *The Problem of Mental Disorder*, New York: McGraw-Hill, 1934.

24. C. Nachin, 'Psychiatrie, sociologie et politique à l'évolution psychiatrique (1925–1960)', *Evolution psychiatrique*, 1976, 41, 43–71.

25. C.F. Nasse, 'Zeitschrift für psychische Arzte: Preface to the first issue', *History of Psychiatry*, 1990, 1, part 2, no. 2: 233–43.

26. J. Postel, 'Une tentative à méditer. Histoire de la première revue française de psychologie médicale 1897–1901', *Psychologie Médicale*, 1971, 3: 645–56.

27. I.W. Riley, 'Mental healing in America', *American Journal of Insanity*, 1910, LXVI: 351–63.

28. G. Ryle, *The Concept of Mind*, London: Hutchinson's University Library, 1949, p. 323.

29. J.A. Ryle, 'The Hippocratic Ideal', *Lancet*, 1934, ii: 1263–5.

30. J. Sibbold, 'Psychiatry in general hospitals', *Review of Neurology and Psychiatry*, 1903, 1: 4–12.

31. C.L. Williams and J. Westermeyer, 'Public health aspects of mental health: the last 75 years of the American Journal of Public Health', *American Journal of Public Health*, 1985, 75: 722–6.

32. F.B. Winslow, Preface, *Journal of Psychological Medicine*, 1845, 1, iii.

33. F.B. Winslow, 'The psychological vocation of the physician', *Journal of Psychological Medicine*, 1854, 7: 106–50.

34. E. von Feuchtersleben, *The Principles of Medical Psychology*, trans. H. Evans Lloyd, London: Sydenham Society, 1847.

11

The medical journals and the politics of public health 1918–90

Jane Lewis

Debates about twentieth-century medicine have been characterized above all by an increased preoccupation with the delivery of health care services. Underlying this preoccupation has been the fundamental assumption that personal health care delivered by a doctor to a patient, whether in the home or in a hospital, is a worthy endeavour that should be widely available. The belief in the progressive power of scientific medicine to cure has been largely shared by policymakers and consumers, as well as by the medical profession itself. In turn, this belief has sustained the view first, that doctors are the best people to determine the content of medical services and second, that developments in medical care should be made available to as many people as possible. The latter view has necessarily involved greater collective effort and a larger role for the state. It is only very recently that faith in the capacity of the medical profession and state medical services has begun to falter. During the 1980s, support for the medical profession in its task of making us healthier and for an increasing role for the state in making medical services more widely available has been questioned.

While the twentieth century has thus been marked by an overarching consensus as to the value of scientific medicine, below this there has nevertheless been considerable room for conflict. The interests of the three major groups of protagonists – the medical profession, 'consumers' and the state – have often differed, and these conflicts have become of paramount importance when faith in the medical profession and in the role of the state in providing medical care are called into question. In particular, while doctors are imbued with 'an absolutist ethic of treatment',[1] the concern of policymakers has been distinctly utilitarian and state provision has been accompanied by a belief in the ability of medical care to work for the collective and not merely the individual good. Thus public expenditure on health care has often been justified in terms of improving the national health and hence national efficiency. None of the three major interest groups is monolithic and this chapter focuses particularly on the different interests of public health doctors from those of general practitioners and hospital doctors.

Public health doctors were and are the smallest of the three major groups of doctors and throughout this century have been struggling both for improved status and a firmer definition of their role. Before the setting up of the National Health Service (NHS) public health doctors found themselves to be in something of an impossible position. As increasing importance was attached to clinical medicine and the individual patient/doctor relationship, they were not uncommonly referred to disparagingly as the 'drains doctors'. But when they began, in the early twentieth century, to develop what was called 'personal preventive medicine', then they risked treading on the toes of the general practitioner. They were additionally suspect because of their positions as salaried employees of local government, a status the independent general practitioner was determined to avoid. The divide between public health and other doctors was therefore large and it is not surprising to find that when conflict arose the *British Medical Journal* (*BMJ*) pursued a consistent line of support for the majority group of general practitioners.

Public health had its own journals, *Public Health* and the independent *Medical Officer.* These took up the cudgels on behalf of the specialty when necessary against the British Medical Association (BMA) and the *BMJ*, but their opposition was always muted not least by the reliance that public health doctors placed on the BMA for help in salary negotiations. On the whole, the public health journals adopted a reactive stance. Different views as to what public health practice consisted of were published, but the views of the editors of these journals were, like those of the specialty's leaders, constrained by the changing structures for the delivery of health care services. Public health was thus conceived of as a number of tasks that waxed with the passing of certain local government Acts, especially that of 1929, and waned with the introduction of the NHS.

Public health doctors lacked both the vision and the power to challenge the dominance achieved by clinical medicine.

If during the first half of the century the work of public health doctors was generally regarded with considerable suspicion outside the specialty's own journals, after 1948 the position of public health was largely ignored until the 1974 reorganization of the NHS and the establishment of the new specialty, community medicine. Yet the challenge posed by public health – most forcefully perhaps in the 1940s with the setting up of social medicine departments in the universities and again in the 1980s, with the campaign for 'healthy public policy' and the 'new public health' – has arguably been fundamental to the question 'whither medicine', traditionally beloved by leader writers in medical journals.

During the last fifteen years, evidence that medical services may have little to do with health status has grown more insistent, such that the power of scientific medicine and the beneficial consequences of meeting the never-ending demand for it have become contested rather than shared ideas. Policymakers have responded to social scientists' and health economists' questions as to scientific medicine's ability to deliver health, first by seeking to exert greater control over decision-making (and hence over doctors) and thereby to shift resources away from the expensive acute care sector and towards community care; and second by managing health services more efficiently, which has entailed the exploration of alternatives to the state's involvement in delivering services. In pursuing these new strategies, government has sought an alliance with the patient or 'consumer', who should, it argues, be allowed greater choice in health care. Despite the apparent willingness of policymakers to address the issue of the content of medical care and the position of the consumer for the first time, the policy response has been dictated primarily by concerns over costs. In this climate, the demands of many public health doctors for a broad intersectoral approach to health promotion and to prevention may acquire new relevance. In this regard, it is significant that the rather narrowly based review of the specialty carried out by a committee chaired by the Chief Medical Officer, Donald Acheson, has received strong criticism from within the specialty which has been published in the leader columns of the *BMJ*, the first time that the journal has taken a lead in stimulating debate about the role of public health.

The increasing importance of personal health care and the role of public health in the early twentieth century

The focus of nineteenth-century health policy was preeminently environmental: all dirt was considered dangerous.[2] By the end of the century, social investigators were convinced that physical well-being was a necessary prerequisite for further social progress. The nineteenth-century vision of health policy was convincingly broad. In particular, the public health Acts were permitted to serve as a filter for more general social reform. Typically, major public health Acts were also housing Acts. As Anthony Sutcliffe has perceptively argued, the 'urban variable' acted as a spur to state intervention because a large number of social questions concerned with poverty and housing as well as health were packed into the fear of urban degeneration and physical deterioration.[3] The urban environment was feared to be producing a race of degenerates, physically stunted and morally inferior. The slippage between social and moral categories, so characteristic of Victorian social science, only served to intensify fear of contamination. Fear, together with religious zeal and civic pride (albeit often moderated by ratepayer parsimony), combined to produce the sanitary reform associated with nineteenth-century health reform.

The images of early twentieth-century debates about health and ideas for reform are rather different and are indicative of the growing emphasis on personal health care that was legitimated by scientific advances, particularly in bacteriology. Once it was realized that dirt *per se* did not cause infectious disease, the broad mandate of public health to deal with all aspects of environmental sanitation and housing as the means of promoting cleanliness disappeared. In Starr's words, the concept of dirt 'narrowed', thereby also proving considerably cheaper to clean up.[4] Increasingly, emphasis was placed on what the individual should do to ensure personal hygiene. The campaign to reduce infant mortality provides an especially clear example of this approach. The campaign to 'glorify, dignify and purify' motherhood began in earnest after the Boer War. Epidemiological studies of the problem, conducted in the late 1900s by medical officers of health employed by local authority public health departments, revealed the death rate to be highest in poor inner city slums, yet government officials and public health doctors tended to view maternal and child welfare in terms of a series of discrete personal health problems, to be solved by the provision of health visitors, infant welfare centres and better maternity services. Before the First World War, the bulk of their attention was focused on health education, encouraging mothers to breast feed and strive for higher standards of domestic hygiene. Clinic work was seen as 'applied physiology', a new kind of personal preventive clinical medicine.[5]

In 1908, the editor of *Public Health* reflected on the shift towards a concern with personal preventive medicine and on the way in which it was 'generally acknowledged' that modern public health work was the province of the pathologist and the physician rather than the sanitary engineer. Increasingly, it seemed, public health was concerned with the application of general principles to individual personal differences:

> the most effective work is that which is individualised, and the consideration of the individual human unit will become a matter of increasing importance in our system of public health administration, with the increase and development in that system of the work of the physician.[6]

This view of the work of public health was broadly supported by public health doctors and given special prominence by Sir George Newman, Chief Medical Officer to the Board of Education and from 1919 to the new Ministry of Health, in a series of memoranda, pamphlets and books. He insisted that public health was no longer primarily concerned with sewerage, disinfection, the suppression of nuisances, the notification and registration of disease and the implementation of bye-law regulations, but rather was about 'the domestic, social and personal life of the people'.[7] It was therefore necessary for the public health doctor to have personal contact with the individual in order to provide health education. In his memorandum on the practice of preventive medicine, first issued in 1919, he argued for a new 'synthesis and integration' in medicine and, in particular, a closer integration between preventive and curative medicine. He was convinced that 'the whole science and art of preventive medicine is . . . essentially clinical in origin and purpose' and he emphasized the importance of a clinical training for MOsH.[8]

The Times attacked Newman's ideas as 'socialistic', preferring the proposals of the Dawson Report on medical and allied services (published in 1919), which was explicit in making the general practitioner the key figure in its scheme for the delivery of medical services and which advocated passing to the GP the personal preventive services that were being developed by the local authorities.[9] However, the *BMJ* supported both, perceiving that the essence of Newman's thought was a commitment to the power of preventive medicine as health education, not a belief in state medicine as *The Times* feared. The *BMJ* had fought hard against the 1909 Minority Report to the Royal Commission on the Poor Laws (authored by Sidney and Beatrice Webb), which favoured passing poor law medicine to the public health departments, because it feared that this would lead in the direction of a free service.[10] The journal had also expressed considerable relief when the Edwardian debate on the structure for delivering health care services was resolved in favour of a scheme of national insurance, which did not propose to create a special class of whole-time medical officers, but rather to enrol the GP as an independent practitioner.[11] In 1918, the journal welcomed Sir George Newman's memorandum on medical education to the president of the Board of Education as 'epoch-making' and in particular hailed Newman's emphasis on the GP as 'the foundation of medicine' in Britain.[12]

Newman continued to insist on the importance of the GP's independent status, which satisfied the BMA and the *BMJ*,[13] but in terms of practical medical politics, public health doctors had good reason to feel that their position was strengthening, largely because of the increase in tasks allotted to the public health departments during the inter-war years. During this period, governments failed to extend health service provision under the National Health Insurance Act and instead added piecemeal to services provided by the local authorities via the public health departments. By 1939, local authorities were permitted to provide maternal and child welfare services, including obstetrical and gynaecological specialist treatment; a school medical service, including clinics treating minor ailments; dentistry; school meals and milk; TB schemes involving sanatorium treatment, clinics and aftercare services; health centres, the most elaborate being that built by the Finsbury Borough Council in 1938; and had responsibility for developing local regional cancer schemes. The most important addition to the medical officer of health's responsibility came in 1929 when local authorities were permitted to take over administration of the poor law hospitals, and medical officers of health found themselves taking on the role of medical superintendent.

Thus from a position of growing strength, in terms of the tasks they were being called upon to perform, MOsH spoke with increasing confidence of the importance of the public health service in leading the way in preventive medicine, primarily through the work of educating the public in personal hygiene, and of the importance of educating the GP to play his part. Throughout the 1920s, public health departments were able to sustain their claim that public health work was mainly clinical medicine, but clinical medicine of a special kind, by following the principles of Newman. The division of labour between MOsH and GPs rested on the separation of health education and advice from treatment. The evidence suggests that public health departments were, in fact, careful not to offer any treatment other than for the mildest ailments, but the boundary between the two types of provision was obviously hard to draw and indeed was sustained largely by a system of health services in which treatment was not free at the point of access. Philosophically, public health had boxed itself into a rather narrow corner that was hard to distinguish from 'curative' medicine.

Indeed, during the 1920s, GPs continually raised the spectre of 'encroachment' by public health doctors on their private practices. In 1921 the *BMJ* called attention to this issue in a leader that criticized Willesden's Public Health Department for offering medical treatment to mothers and children without restrictions as to income.[14] In 1928 Dr A. Cox, the secretary of the BMA, was asked to investigate and report on the issue. While favouring the cause of the GP, he argued judiciously that 'we would be doing a great service to the profession if we educated them [GPs] to claim and to take their part in the present scheme, instead of bemoaning the encroachments on private practice'.[15] Cox pointed out that the local authority services for mothers, infants and school children had grown out of the Medical Inspection of School Children Act 1907, which the BMA had supported, and that the Ministry, and in particular Newman, had never denied the importance of the role played by the GP in the medical services. Cox observed local authority work in six areas and concluded that 'few private practitioners . . . have any first hand knowledge of the procedure. I was astounded, on asking the doctors I met at various meetings to find that hardly any had ever been inside one of these centres'.[16] In short, GPs had shown little inclination to do work that all were agreed should be done. In every area that he visited, Cox was impressed by the genuine attempt that was made to get the patient to consult a private doctor before giving anything except treatment for very minor ailments. Cox limited his recommendations to a plea that MOsH should employ more part-time GPs in clinics in order to enlist the GP in the cause of preventive medicine and to promote harmony in the profession.

However, the BMA's Committee on Encroachments on the Sphere of Private Practice by the Activities of Local Authorities, to which Cox passed his report, took a much firmer line. In its Interim Report, issued in 1928, the Committee urged private practitioners not to allow personal preventive work 'to pass without protest' to local authority doctors.[17] Its Final Report stated firmly that medical practice with individuals, whether sick or requiring knowledge on how to maintain their health, 'naturally belongs to, because it is best provided by, private practitioners'.[18] The Committee claimed that the private GP had a wider range of clinical experience and a more direct knowledge of home conditions than the medical officer. It concluded by recommending a complete separation between the world of GPs and MOsH in much the same manner as the Dawson Report: 'The main sphere of the private practitioner is the giving of medical advice and treatment to individuals; the main sphere of the public health medical officer is the promotion of healthy conditions for the community'.[19] While stressing that the MOH and the GP should take an interest in each other's work, the Committee recommended that public health doctors should not undertake any clinical work that could be done by a GP. This amounted to a direct refutation by the BMA of public health's claim to be doing 'applied physiology', as the *Medical Officer* called it in 1930.[20]

The response from public health doctors was muted. The *Medical Officer* published an angry editorial in which it argued that the term 'encroachment' was incorrect; local authorities were merely undertaking work in fields that the GP failed to occupy.[21] It also disputed the idea that only GPs possessed enough knowledge about the family situation of the individual to undertake preventive work and defended the employment of full-time medical officers in clinics. Nevertheless, the journal ended by endorsing the idea that GPs should do clinic work where possible. In fact MOsH did not have to be overly defensive. As the *Medical Officer* pointed out, so-called encroachment was sanctioned by law.[22] Indeed, in 1929, MOsH were preoccupied with the implications of the Local Government Act which further enlarged their empire by giving them control over what had been the poor law hospitals, and to which they preferred to appoint consultants rather than GPs.[23] Dr Buchan, the MOH for Willesden, where the wide range of personal medical services provided by the local authority had roused particular ire among GPs, was led to remark that 'the very large provisions and concentrations in respect of public health and medical work made by the Local Government Act of 1929 are likely to lead to a State Medical Service'.[24]

Despite this further consolidation of the position of public health departments, the status of the MOH remained low within the medical profession and, paradoxically, MOsH were reliant on the support of the BMA in respect to salary negotiations. In 1923, the BMA and the Society of Medical Officers of Health agreed on a scheme of cooperation whereby the BMA agreed to support a minimum salary scale for public health doctors, and both organizations altered their constitutions to allow direct representation by the other on their respective governing bodies.[25] In return, the Society of Medical Officers of Health agreed that it would not act independently on medico-political matters. The agreement was welcomed by the *Medical Officer* as promoting harmony in the profession,[26] but it undoubtedly helped to stifle the voice of the public health doctor. The agreement was renegotiated periodically during the 1920s and 1930s, but its terms continued to be controversial. One MOH wrote in outrage that the society had 'been sold body and soul to the British Medical Association'.[27] MOsH in the East Midland Branch of the Society observed correctly that the BMA did not see fit to consult the Society in framing its views on 'A General Medical Service for the Nation', published in 1937, which again promoted the cause of the independent GP at the expense of the salaried medical officer.[28]

During the 1930s, as medical officers of health expanded their work of health administration in respect of the municipal hospitals, the Society of Medical Officers of Health confidently predicted that public health doctors would soon control the medical services, which flew in the face of the BMA's implacable opposition to a salaried service controlled by local government. The *Medical Officer* expressed some concern as to whether the kind of work being performed by public health doctors during the 1930s, particularly in hospital administration, had not diverted them from their central task of prevention, warning MOsH not to neglect the work of 'individual prevention', that was still in its infancy according to the president of the Society of Medical Officers of Health, in favour of 'pathology'.[29] At the Public Health Congress of 1930, Sir Arthur Newsholme, who had been the Chief Medical Officer to the Local Government Board before the First World War, suggested that the work of co-ordinating the medical services was an inevitable result of the 1929 Local Government Act, but would prove a temporary phenomenon.[30] But the editor of the *Medical Officer* wondered, more realistically perhaps, whether MOsH would be able easily to return 'from the pursuit of pathology to their proper allegiance to physiology',[31] commenting crossly: 'Much recent public health work seems to aim at converting it into a gigantic hospital'.[32] The *Medical Officer* insisted that, while the responsibilities of the public health department encompassed sanitation, treatment and adminstration, as well as prevention, the MOH should devote most of his time to the latter. Clearly, prevention was still being defined after the manner of Newman. As late as 1937, the journal reiterated that 90 per cent of the medical officer's job was clinical, but in the sense of 'applied physiology' rather than the provision of treatment.[33]

There is no evidence that the philosophy of public health developed further in the 1930s, or that the *Medical Officer*'s concern regarding the hospital responsibilities of MOsH was widely shared. Little on this theme surfaced in *Public Health* and at least one MOH produced a spirited defence of the MOH's involvement in hospitals as being very much a part of preventive work.[34] However, recent work has suggested the extent to which the public health doctor neglected his traditional role as watchdog over the people's health, particularly with regard to questions of nutrition standards and the effect of high mass unemployment on health status.[35] To this extent, the *BMJ*'s charge that MOsH were guilty of doing work that was the province of other specialties, and in so doing failing to develop their own agendas, was not without foundation.

The majority of MOsH were content to expand the range of services provided by their public health departments, expecting that the balance of medical care provision would soon swing in favour of a state service, whereupon the MOH as the only salaried doctor would come into his own. However, not only did the BMA remain resolutely opposed to such a vision, favouring the extension of national health insurance and a central role for the GP, but the Ministry of Health showed no inclination towards either an extension of insurance or a fully fledged state salaried service. For all Newman's willingness to add in an *ad hoc* manner to the powers of local authorities, he was not prepared to argue that the balance of medical care provision should be swung in favour of the public health service. It was this that rendered public health doctors' apparent willingness to allow the content and direction of public health to be defined by its tasks; a fragile basis for future prosperity.

In 1946, the National Health Service Act removed the municipal hospital from the purview of the MOH and by making the GP service accessible to all also eroded the rationale for the local authority clinics. MOsH were left to bewail 'the remnants' that remained. The president of the Society of Medical Officers of Health, J. Johnstone Jervis, felt that the only hope lay in the development of health centres but, of course, this did not occur until the late 1960s.[36] The *Medical Officer* tried to strike a positive note when it remarked that the MOH would at last be free of his hospital administration duties, and would be able to devote himself to 'epidemiology'.[37] The journal added that the responsibilities for hospital administration had in all probability diverted MOsH from the business of prevention, which accounted for 'the "discovery" of social medicine, which had for a century been the daily work of the MOH'.[38] The *Medical Officer*'s comment on the reasons for public health's failure to become involved in social medicine may well have been accurate, but the public health journals had proved essentially dismissive of this important wartime effort to revitalize public health, and this was to leave the specialty without a firm sense of direction in the post-NHS world.

The *BMJ* published Sir Farquhar Buzzard's endorsement of social medicine in 1942 in which he described centres for social medicine undertaking research in the promotion and preservation of health, coordinating social and health services and encouraging the reorientation of the medical curriculum.[39] In its editorial column, the journal welcomed the subsequent setting up of the Institute for Social Medicine at Oxford and noted approvingly its clinical orientation: 'This imaginative move has not had its origin in the public health service or in the Government Department officially concerned with health'.[40] The first professor of social medicine at Oxford, John Ryle, followed Buzzard with a letter to the *BMJ* in which he attempted to flesh out his definition of social medicine as 'applied aetiology':

> Social medicine is clinical medicine activated in its aetiological inquiries by social conscience as well as scientific interest and having as its main purpose the education of progressive and lay thought and the direction of legislation on behalf of national health and efficiency.[41]

This was Ryle's first attempt at a definition of social medicine and it neatly encapsulated the two most important building blocks in his thinking on the subject, the importance of social conscience and a commitment to clinical medicine. It seems that, by the late 1940s, the latter had become the more important strand. An editorial in *The Lancet* also deemed it appropriate that social medicine should have grown out of hospital medicine rather than public health, while acknowledging that the new social medicine experts would probably require 'some of the public health techniques such as field studies and the applications of statistics'.[42] The public health journals reacted by denying that there was anything new in social medicine and by deploring its high academic tone. The *Medical Officer* was especially scathing in its review of the report of the Oxford Institute on its work between 1943 and 1950, accusing it of ignoring the contribution of public health and describing its account of the introduction of social medicine as 'naive'. The journal was particularly incensed by the Institute's attack on the value of mass radiography and infant welfare clinics.[43] Thus social medicine became alienated from the practice of public health, but at the same time it failed to have the kind of impact on the medical schools that Buzzard and Ryle had hoped for. Most schools reacted by slightly modifying their departments of public health, but without fundamentally changing their approach to medical education. Furthermore, a dangerous schism developed between social medicine academics and public health practitioners which contributed to public health's isolation in the post-war world.

From public health to community medicine and back again

The immediate inclination of MOsH and public health departments after the implementation of the NHS Act in 1948 was not to take up the suggestion of the *Medical Officer* and of at least one professor of preventive medicine that they engage more seriously with epidemiology and the business of prevention,[44] but rather to look for new services to administer, especially under section 28 of the NHS Act, which referred to the possibility of providing welfare services for preventing illness, helping those suffering from illness, or for providing aftercare services.

Responsibility for running ambulance services, home helps and old people's homes became particularly time-consuming tasks. As a result, local authorities associations expressed the view that MOsH were but 'administrators with medical knowledge', implying that they had no connection with the mainstream of medicine and were fulfilling a largely executive function. Public health doctors spent much of the 1950s and 1960s fighting the insistence of local authorities that they should be paid on a scale comparable to other administrative officers rather than to other doctors, and coping with the hierarchical nature of the public health service which was closer to the rather rigid workings of the unreformed local government system than to the medical profession. The public image of the MOH was unhappily personified in the dreary and obstructionist character of Dr Snoddy in the popular television series, 'Dr Finlay's Casebook', which was concerned with the daily work of a general practitioner.

Within the specialty, debate centred on whether public health doctors should devote themselves more wholeheartedly to the work of medical administration. Professor J.N. Morris, who was a leading proponent of social medicine and was to be influential in formulating the role of the community physician, argued in a Chadwick Trust Lecture in 1957 that prevention and cure should be integrated in the work of the GP.[45] Many medical officers of health agreed that the days of the clinical medical officer were numbered. Certainly the *Medical Officer* saw something rather attractive in the prospect of the GP taking over the clinical work, and wondered if this would not then allow the MOH to emerge 'as a coordinator and overseer of the health services of his community', rather than being 'confined to the administration of the smallest part of them'.[46]

From the early 1960s, it was obvious that academics, central government and senior public health doctors were not convinced that a firm base could be built for public health that included clinical work. In an influential article on the future of the family doctor, published at the height of the 'crisis' over general practice, Titmuss fuelled debate about the future of the MOH by asking whether, if the GP became more of a community doctor, there would still be a place for the MOH.[47] Dr J.J.A. Reid, the MOH for Northamptonshire, immediately replied that the answer was to train the MOH in medical administration and transform him into a specialist whose knowledge and techniques would be available to his colleagues in all branches of medicine. Reid wanted to make the MOH 'a broad adviser' to the health services.[48] Reid was exceptional among MOsH in taking up the call for a new training and a new role; he went on to become a leading advocate of community medicine and the community physician. Many MOsH were dissatisfied with the training provided by the diploma in public health,[49] but there was no overwhelmingly enthusiastic response to the new focus on medical administration. Administration continued to be understood by most in terms of organization and methods.

The *BMJ* offered very little comment on public health matters during the 1950s. But, beginning in the early 1960s, it urged the need to unite public health with the other parts of the NHS, observing that the 'chronic ills' of the specialty were due to 'belonging to two worlds and getting the best of neither'.[50] The *BMJ* played no significant role in the reconceptualization of public health as community medicine. Its lack of attention to the role of public health was reflected in its reaction to the recommendations of the Seebohm Committee on local authority and allied personal social services. The BMA proposed to the Committee the fusing of the health and welfare departments under the MOH, which represented a traditional defence of the medical model that was quite out of sympathy with the mood of the Committee including its only medical member, J.N. Morris, who, like his fellow committee member and co-operator, Richard Titmuss, was convinced that MOsH were unable to articulate any sound principle for their involvement in welfare work. Titmuss had floated the idea of unified social service departments to a medical audience at the Royal Society of Health Congress in 1965,[51] but neither MOsH nor the BMA took note of the influential arguments of social scientists regarding trends in social services during the 1960s, which left them at a considerable disadvantage in understanding the rapid movement in health and social services at the end of the decade.

In 1970, the *BMJ* noted with alarm the serious drop in the number of UK students taking the DPH, from 87 in 1963–4 to 43 in 1968–9, and urged other specialties to extend 'tangible support' to their beleaguered public health colleagues.[52] When the establishment of a faculty of community medicine was announced in 1971, the journal welcomed it unreservedly, promoting the role of the new community physician as someone 'committed to the measurement, planning and development of all services for the prevention and treatment of disease in each administrative area' without whose work 'an integrated health service cannot be achieved'.[53] But the journal offered no further analysis of the way in which the community physician's role was being envisaged or implemented.

It was J.N. Morris who first defined the role of the community physician. He believed strongly that public health practice should be grounded more firmly in the principles of modern epidemiology. His extremely influential monograph on epidemiology identified the major uses of the subject as historical study, community diagnosis, analysis of the workings of health services, analysis of individual risks and changes, the identification of syndromes and the completion of the clinical picture.[54] From this he evolved the concept of a community physician responsible for community diagnosis and thus providing the 'intelligence' necessary for efficiency and effective administration of the health services.[55]

But it would seem that the *BMJ*'s and policymakers' understanding of the role of the community physician differed in emphasis from that of academics. The key documents published prior to NHS reorganization in 1974 saw the new community physician as the key to effective integration of the health services, linking lay administrators to clinicians and coordinating the work of the NHS with that of the local authorities. The community physician was recognized as a specialist adviser, with particular skills in epidemiology, but a substantial number of community physicians were to be given management responsibilities in the new consensus management teams in order to utilize their expertise properly.[56] It seems clear that, while the faculty of community medicine stressed the community physician's specialist adviser role and stressed the complementarity between community and clinical medicine, policymakers stressed the importance of the community physician recommending changes in the deployment of resources and of management.

By 1974, the *BMJ* was expressing considerable dissatisfaction with the practice of community medicine, while offering little by way of constructive comment:

> At first sight it seems difficult to see what common ground exists for medical administrators, public health doctors, and academics from departments of social medicine. Too often those asking for explanations have been fobbed off with talk about management expertise and coordination – a word-salad of jargon.[57]

This did not give any recognition to the extraordinarily difficult position community physicians found themselves in.

MOsH moved into the role of community physician believing that they were to be the linchpins of the new NHS, coordinating and administering services, but with little idea as to the meaning of their formal role in the new management structure or the place of 'management' in their total package of tasks and concerns. From the beginning, community physicians found the 'community hat' a difficult one to wear. The 1968 Todd Commission on Medical Education had proposed that the term community should embrace the whole population, including those in institutions,[58] but increasingly 'community' came to describe the non-hospital services. Thus, while it was intended that the community physician should provide the necessary 'intelligence' for adjudicating the resource needs of various types of health services, including the hospital, in practice the title of community physician often meant that other members of the management teams expected him to speak for the community services outside the hospital. On the other hand, the battle to come to terms with the problems of the hospital services meant that many community physicians who continued to feel considerable commitment to the extra-hospital health services, and to the work of prevention and promotion, felt that their work was determined more by the needs of the NHS than those of the communities they served.[59] Thus the position of community physicians was subject to serious conflicts in terms of both their relationship with other members of the medical profession, and the nature of their primary responsibility, whether for the management of health services or for the analysis of health problems and health needs. The image of the community physician as primarily a part of the NHS management structure was reinforced when in 1976 community medicine posts were included in a review of management costs, and as severe financial restraints were imposed on the NHS, the position of the community physician became increasingly difficult.

During the 1980s, as integration of the health service ceased to be the focus of government's attention and as the concept of management shifted away from the achievement of consensus towards a more straightforward preoccupation with careful administration and clear lines of accountability, so less attention was paid to the role of community medicine in policy documents. The 1979 government document which signalled the 1982 NHS reorganization made no mention of the specialty and the emphasis was clearly on better management of the hospitals.[60] The Griffiths Report of 1983 also focused firmly on the hospitals and recommended the appointment of a single general manager, readily identifiable at all levels of administration. Because the role of the community physician was determined in large part by the place he occupied in the 1974 NHS structure, this shift had clear implications for the specialty. While the tensions between the community physician's role as specialist adviser or manager have largely disappeared since 1984 – very few community physicians became general managers – so also have the tasks of community medicine become fragmented and the numbers of community physicians have been reduced in many districts.

These changes in the fortunes of community medicine should be located more widely. The reorganization of the NHS in 1974 was motivated in large part by the Treasury's desire to gain more control over public spending by the DHSS. In this attempt, the community physician was perceived by policy-makers as the linchpin. When costs in the hospital sector continued to rise, further reorganizations followed and in 1984 professional managers rather than community physicians were seen as the answer to containing costs and achieving a more rational allocation of resources. In all this, it would appear that government has effectively overlooked the other side of community medicine's tasks, that of preventing disease and promoting health through the provision of specialist advice. Government in the 1980s was not oblivious to the idea of prevention and promotion, although it was not inclined to link it either to the need for a body of specialist medical practitioners, or to the need for collective provision, as was shown by the poor response to the Black Report on Inequalities in Health.[61]

One of the reasons that governments have gained confidence in their dealings with the medical profession is the publicity accorded to studies which suggest that medical services have played very little part in raising the health status of populations.[62] In the light of such evidence, governments have tried first to switch resources away from the expensive acute sector to preventive medicine, community care and the 'cinderella' specialties and in so doing have harnessed the rhetoric of prevention to the cause of cost control. When proponents of social medicine talked about prevention in the 1940s, they meant the identification of social and environmental factors inimical to health. However, the concept of prevention in the last decade has concentrated on the responsibility to maintain a healthy lifestyle. Second, governments have sought to invoke the right of consumers to increased choice and have sought to achieve this negatively, by decreasing the power of providers rather than by empowering consumers.[63]

Because community medicine was embedded in the structure of the NHS it can be argued that it requires political will to revitalize the specialty. But current government thinking is along very different lines from that of 1974 and the role of community medicine does not figure largely on the political agenda. The government enquiry into the future development of the 'public health function', published in 1988[64] was prompted by the failure to respond adequately to two outbreaks of communicable disease. In recommending a return to 'public health medicine' and greater emphasis on the prevention of communicable disease, the enquiry's report may be read as an attempt to retrench and to secure a separate but firm niche for public health within the NHS. What seems to be significantly different from the early 1970s is that those within the specialty who would seek to use the new positions of director of public health at district and regional level to broaden the mandate of public health in line with the promotion of 'healthy public policy' are now being provided with a platform in the *BMJ*.[65] Perhaps for the first time the debate about public health, which has significant political and medico-political implications, is taking place in this journal.

Notes

1. R. Klein, *The Politics of the NHS*, London: Longman, 1983.
2. Paul Starr, *The Social Transformation of American Medicine*, New York: Basic Books, 1982, p. 189.
3. A. Sutcliffe, 'In search of the urban variable', in D. Fraser and A. Sutcliffe (eds) *The Pursuit of Urban History*, London: Arnold, 1983.
4. Starr, *Social Transformation of American Medicine*, p. 189.
5. For further discussion of this concept, see J. Lewis, *What Price Community Medicine?* Brighton: Wheatsheaf, 1986.
6. 'The functions of the doctor in public health administration', *Public Health*, 1908, 21: 89.
7. George Newman, *The Foundation of National Health*, London: Ministry of Health, 1928.
8. Ministry of Health, *An Outline of the Practice of Preventive Medicine*, Memorandum by Sir George Newman, London: HMSO, 1926, paras 43–50; and George Newman, *Recent Advances in Medical Education in England*, Memorandum to the Ministry of Health, London: HMSO, 1923, p. 156.
9. 'Health services', editorial, *Public Health*, 1921, 34: 159.
10. 'The Poor Law Commission and medical reform', editorial, *BMJ*, 1909, II: 361.
11. 'The National Insurance Scheme', editorial, *BMJ*, 1911, I: 1134.
12. 'Medical Education in England', editorial, *BMJ*, 1918, II: 117–18.
13. Sir George Newman, 'Preventive medicine and the Ministry of Health', *BMJ*, 1920, II: 635.
14. 'Public health and private practice', editorial, *BMJ*, 1921, I: 908–9.
15. 'Report by Medical Secretary on investigation into the operation of maternal and child welfare centres and school clinics in certain areas', *BMJ*, 1928, II Supplement: 194.
16. ibid., p. 190.
17. 'BMA's Private Practice Committee's Interim Report on Encroachments on the Sphere of Private Practice by the Activities of Local Authorities', *BMJ*, 1928, II Supplement: 185–96.

18. 'Report on Encroachments on the Sphere of Private Practice', *BMJ*, 1929, II: 130.

19. ibid., p. 132.

20. 'Preventive medicine and health insurance', editorial, *Medical Officer*, 1930, 44: 199.

21. 'Encroachments on private practice', editorial, *Medical Officer*, 1929, 41: 31.

22. 'Health authorities and private medical practice', editorial, *Medical Officer*, 1928, 40: 217.

23. Frank Honigsbaum, *The Division in British Medicine*, London: Kogan Page, 1979, p. 138.

24. G. Buchan, 'British public health and its present trend', *Public Health*, 1931, 45: 9.

25. 'Scale of minimum commencing salaries for public health medical officers', *BMJ*, 1923, I Supplement: 151–8; and 'Cooperation with the Society of Medical Officers of Health, *BMJ*, 1923, II Supplement: 35–41.

26. 'The Society of Medical Officers of Health and the BMA', *Medical Officer*, 1923, 30: 87.

27. Letter from W.G. Booth, MOH for Lincolnshire, printed in the editorial col. *Public Health*, 1939, 52: 89.

28. Society of Medical Officers of Health Archives, Wellcome Unit, Oxford, A12, Minutes of the Council of the Society, 17/2/39.

29. 'Medicine and the state', editorial, *Medical Officer*, 1930, 44: 245; and 'The present state of preventive medicine', editorial, *Medical Officer*, 1933, 50: 21.

30. 'Medicine and the state', *Medical Officer*, 1930, 44: 245.

31. ibid.

32. 'Preventive medicine in 1930', editorial, *Medical Officer*, 1931, 45: 1.

33. 'The public health service', editorial, *Medical Officer*, 1937, 58: 95.

34. J. Ferguson, 'Hospital policy in relation to preventive medicine', *Public Health*, 1938, 51: 239.

35. For example, Charles Webster, 'Healthy or hungry thirties?' *History Workshop Journal*, 1982, no. 13: 110–29.

36. J. Johnstone Jervis, 'Has public health any future?' *Public Health*, 1946, 59: 46–9.

37. 'Clinical and preventive medicine', editorial, *Medical Officer*, 1948, 78: 175.

38. 'The MOH and the hospital board', editorial, *Medical Officer*, 1948, 79: 258–9.

39. Sir Farquhar Buzzard, 'The place of social medicine in the reorganisation of health services', *BMJ*, 1942, I: 703–4.

40. 'Social medicine', editorial, *BMJ*, 1942, II: 101.

41. J.A. Ryle, letter, *BMJ*, 1942, II: 801.

42. 'Social pathology', editorial, *Lancet*, 1947, I: 413.

43. 'The Oxford Institute of Social Medicine', editorial, *Medical Officer*, 1951, 85: 12.

44. F. Grundy, 'New paths for public health', *Public Health*, 1953, 63: 190–2.

45. 'Medical care', editorial, *Medical Officer*, 1957, 97: 104.

46. 'Towards a measure of care', editorial, *Medical Officer*, 1962, 108: 93.

47. R.M. Titmuss, 'The role of the family doctor today in the context of Britain's social services', *Lancet*, 1965, I: 2.

48. J.J.A. Reid, 'A new public health – the problems and the challenge', *Public Health*, 1965, 79: 183–96.

49. E.g., R.W. Elliott, MOH for the West Riding. See 'Altering the public health structure', editorial, *Medical Officer*, 1967, 118: 198.

50. 'Public health dilemmas', editorial, *BMJ*, 1923, I: 419; and 'Public health doctors' conference', editorial, *BMJ*, 1966, I: 877.

51. R.M. Titmuss, 'Social work and social science: a challenge for local government', *Royal Society of Health Journal*, 1966, 86: 19–21.

52. 'Public health', editorial, *BMJ*, 1970, III: 236–7.

53. 'Community medicine', editorial, *BMJ*, 1971, II: 417.

54. J.N. Morris, *The Uses of Epidemiology*, Edinburgh: Livingstone, 1969, first edition 1957.

55. J.N. Morris, 'Tomorrow's community physician', *Lancet*, 1969, II: 811–16.

56. DHSS, *Management Arrangements for the Reorganized NHS*, London: HMSO, 1972, and DHSS, *Report of the Working Party on Medical Administrators*, London: HMSO, 1972.

57. 'What is community medicine?', editorial, *BMJ*, 1974, II: 186–7.

58. PP., 'Report of the Royal Commission on Medical Education', Cmnd. 3569, 1967–8, xxv, p. 569.

59. A. Scott Samuel, 'The politics of health', *Community Medicine*, 1979, 1.

60. DHSS and Welsh Office, *Patients First: Consultative Paper on the Structure of the NHS in England and Wales*, London: HMSO, 1979.

61. P. Townsend and N. Davidson, *Inequalities in Health*, Harmondsworth: Penguin, 1982.

62. Thomas McKeown, *The Modern Rise of Population*, London: Edward Arnold, 1976.

63. Celia Davies, 'Things to come; the NHS in the next decade', *Sociology of Health and Illness*, 1987, 9.

64. PP., *Public Health in England*. The Report of the Committee of Inquiry into the Future Development of the Public Health Function, Cmnd. 289, London: HMSO, 1988.

65. John Ashton, 'Acheson: a missed opportunity for the new public health', editorial, *BMJ*, 1988, I: 231; and John Gabbay, 'The new public health', editorial, *BMJ*, 1988, I: 371–2.

12

The *British Medical Journal*, general practitioners and the state 1840–1990

Julian Tudor Hart

This chapter deals with the relation of the *British Medical Journal* (*BMJ*) to general practitioners (GPs) from 1840 to 1990. I shall concentrate on the relation of GPs to society and the state, a subject of fierce belief and contention throughout these 150 years of the *BMJ*, always rumbling and sometimes erupting through its editorials and correspondence columns.

I see a shape to these 150 years, three distinct eras: a phase of radical reform, in which GPs sought allies from the populations they served; a phase of complacent autonomy within a grudgingly accepted Welfare State, in which medical respectability seemed secured by renunciation of any popular alliance; and our contemporary phase, in which GPs again seek allies among their populations to defend the public services they once opposed against reversion to marketed medical care.

The Poor Law

Like its more radical competitor, *The Lancet*, from its birth as a weekly in 1840 to the end of Ernest Hart's editorship in 1898, the *Journal* and the British Medical Association[1] advocated the right of the poor to receive medical care equally with the rich, and opposed trade in medical care as a marketed commodity. As the *Journal* reported in 1848,

> Such is the nature of medical practice that there never is and never can be any regular market price for medical services. The peer and the cottager, if they have a broken leg or an inflammation of the lungs, require the same

> attendance, the same medicines for their cure; yet they cannot by any possibility pay the same amount of remuneration.[2]

Most people were too poor to provide a mass market for medical care, and the carriage trade was too small and too scattered to support the profession. In an era when the placebo effect, exerted chiefly through time and trouble taken with each case, was the only weapon available, doctors had to believe in what they did. For treatment of the impoverished multitude to be credible, it had to involve time and trouble comparable at least with that commanded by the wealthy few. This was simply not possible if care was paid for in pence by the poor and guineas by the rich.

Care of the multitude depended either on contributory insurance from working men, or from propertied ratepayers through Boards of Guardians under the Poor Law Act of 1834.[3] By 1844, 2,800 GPs, 16 per cent of all medical practitioners, held part-time appointments under the Act. The unpauperized poor, and industrial and some agricultural workers and their families, got their care through medical clubs and the originally small and locally based mutual aid and insurance societies which provided subsistence payments and elementary medical care. Care and medicines were paid for by fixed capitation, from weekly subscriptions or deductions from wages.

Throughout the nineteenth century, the *Journal* provides ample evidence that both employment by Boards of Guardians and Club practice were sweated industries. An example of work under the Poor Law was given by Dr F.S. Garlick in 1847,[4] medical officer for Halifax. He was contracted to the Board of Guardians to serve the poor after assessment of need for care and pauper status by a relieving officer. Under these arrangements he saw an average 14.3 new cases a week, requiring 58 home visits and 313 prescriptions, which he made up and paid for out of his annual salary of £80. This made £1 10s 9d a week, or just over 6 pence per home visit to 'courts, lanes, alleys, cellars, garrets, and crowded lodging houses – places which baffle all description, but which may truly be pronounced sinks of misery, filth, and destitution'.

Paid badly or not at all, GPs under contract to the Poor Law were too close to the demand to avoid responsibility. A notorious case in 1848 was Dr Berncastle, assistant to Dr

Bottomley of Croydon, called to attend a pauper woman in labour.[5] While her friends hunted for the relieving officer, Dr Berncastle paid her three visits. He was then told the order was refused by the parish authorities, and ceased attendance. The woman died from exhaustion. There was an inquest, where the coroner reproved Dr Berncastle for his callousness, followed by this press comment:

> In most of the cases of neglect that have shocked the public for the last few years in consequence of the maladministration of the laws relating to the poor, it has been a remarkable fact that the medical officers concerned have apparently believed that there was nothing in their conduct to warrant the disgust it has elicited . . . a set of unfeeling directors or guardians of the poor have got hold of a medical man as heartless as themselves, and, by keeping each other in countenance, they have all been emboldened to the commission of acts of the most hardened cruelty.[5]

Rejecting such comment in the lay press, the *Journal* suggested the guardians had

> intended to betray their medical officer into a gratuitous attendance on a pauper case, and on his failing to do so, they are themselves solely responsible, not only for the injustice done to him, but for the whole of the mischief which resulted. . . . If the case was a pauper one, the relieving officer and the Board of Guardians were the parties who should have been censured; if not, why is Dr Berncastle's humanity to be called in question, because having already given much, he did not give more? . . . suppose these said twelve jurymen, bakers, spirit dealers, &c., to have been severally informed of this, and roused at midnight for the supply of the necessary food and stimulus, and their wives called upon to come out and administer them on the plea that the woman had no nurse, nor the means of procuring one; would any one of them have bestowed as much attention on the request as Dr Berncastle did to the call upon him? Would they not have said, 'No the public provides for these things! Go to the relieving officer!', and then have closed their doors . . .[5]

GPs earned a pittance attending the poor, but served as scapegoats for flint-hearted philosophers (notably Edwin Chadwick) who deliberately designed the Poor Law to repel all but the most desperate applicants. Doctors risked their own lives. 1848 was the year of the Irish potato famine, prompting the following news item:[6]

> **Mortality of Medical Practitioners in Ireland from Fever**
> Scarcely a week passes without the loss of three or four district medical officers from this cause being announced in the *Dublin Medical Press.* During the late epidemic, of 27 physicians attached to fever hospitals and districts in the province of Ulster, attacked with fever in the course of their duties, 14, or more than half, died, leaving 9 widows and 37 children, for the most part scantily or not at all provided for.

The response today of some doctors to patients with AIDS suggests little understanding of this heritage.

Club practice

Earnings for GPs in contract with clubs and friendly societies generally resembled those paid under the Poor Law. For a whole year's responsibility for each adult male benefit member, the Dorset County Friendly Society in 1848[7] paid its medical officers 2s.6d; for their children over 16 and wives 2s. (excluding childbirth); for the first three children under 16 1s.; and for each additional child 9 pence.[7] All medicines, and all attendances when requested, were to be supplied within these capitation payments. The average annual period of sickness was estimated at just over 6 days, about 30 days a year for a husband, wife and three children, attendance for which worked out at 3 pence a day, covering all medicines and other expenses.

The medical press was preoccupied with problems of club practice until the Insurance Act of 1911 replaced it. The most comprehensive account appeared not in the *BMJ,* but in *The Lancet*'s pamphlet of 1896, the 'Battle of the Clubs'.[8] *The Lancet*'s correspondent travelled throughout the industrial heartlands. Average medical earnings ranged from 9s. a year for male patients earning £1 a week or more, down to 7s. a year for men earning less than 15s.; women were paid for at 4s. a year (excluding childbirth), and children at 3s. a year. In Southampton a quarter of the population was attended under club schemes at 4s. a year per head. Portsmouth Dockyard Medical Benefit Society got its doctors at an annual cost of 2s. 2d each. One GP went through his accounts to show he had made 1,958 visits and conducted 4,650 office consultations for a total income of £38.11s.11d.; 1.4 pence per item of service. On the eve of the Insurance Act, things were getting worse, not better.

GPs were too close to social realities to believe the poor could be served as consumers in a free market. *The Lancet*'s correspondent quoted a general opinion:

> . . . it is better that the miners should belong to clubs, otherwise their medical attendant will get no pay at all. A penny, twopence, even sixpence a week can be obtained without difficulty, but shilling fees or 18-penny fees with medicine included are never paid.

In York he found GPs critical of some of their colleagues who tried to collect economic fees. They gave as example a servant girl who received a medical bill for £15, but 'whose annual wage barely amounted to that sum. Then a bill of perhaps £30 would be presented to the head of a family whose income might not exceed £200'.

Pressure for reform

Throughout the rest of the nineteenth century, the *Journal* reported a steady flow of professional meetings documenting these grievances, and deputations drawing them to the attention of sympathetic members of parliament and ministers, or attempting to drive harder bargains with the increasingly centralized insurance companies which were gradually taking over the mutual aid and friendly societies which financed the clubs.

As with other trades unions and professional pressure groups, the negotiators' only real strength lay in legislative exclusion of unqualified practitioners, and organization of the profession to reduce internal competition through professional solidarity. So long as doctors had to accept all work, however degrading, there was no way to raise the price of their labour.

The arguments of these spokesmen were well documented, modest, self-critical and (in contrast to the next era) accepted the need for accountability and enforcement of standards. For example, in 1848[2] the Committee of Poor Law Medical Convention admitted:

> At present the real amount of responsibility of the medical officer is by no means great. It is true he may often incur great blame for a very trifling cause, or perhaps from no just cause; but he may be guilty of great neglect without its being known to his employers. This arises from the circumstance of Boards of Guardians, however much they may desire to insure good medical attendance to their poor, being unacquainted with medical science, and therefore being really unable to judge whether the amount and quality of the attendance rendered by their medical officer is at all equal to the occasion. In all other public departments in which medical services are required there is a system of inspection by competent medical authorities, which is absolutely necessary to a proper supervision, and which would introduce a real responsibility if it were applied to the Poor Law medical system . . . Such a system of professional inspection is not only necessary to do justice to the poor; it is also necessary to insure justice to the medical officer, for the extent of his services, and the exactness with which he performs his duties can only be appreciated by persons who are thoroughly acquainted with medical science and practice.
>
> It has been objected that the medical profession have the remedy in their own hands; that they need not continue to hold their appointments for which they are so badly paid, but may give them up to others who will be ready to take them. It is true that . . . however low the so-called remuneration may be fixed, there will frequently be found men with the necessary testimonials prepared to take appointments; but these men will in their turn reiterate the same complaints . . . for the grievance will remain, an undue amount of labour, attended with much anxiety and personal risk, will be demanded for an insufficient recompense. The natural result follows; unless an abiding sense of duty and self-respect animates the medical officer, harshness and neglect take the place of kindness and zeal.

This argument was understood by the great and good to whom these petitions were addressed, but they did not share the strange belief of doctors that the poor need at least as much care as the rich. With a permanent surplus of poor doctors available to take appointments, almost nothing was done to change the terms of employment under the Poor Law until the Lloyd George Insurance Act largely superseded it in 1912.

Public health and private practice

Tougher arguments on behalf of authoritarian public health had more success, and were supported by the *Journal* with surprisingly little regard to the contending merits of preventive and curative medicine.

Edwin Chadwick's head was as hard as his heart. Generously reported in the *Journal* in 1847,[9] he showed that conditions for the poor in Liverpool led to 10,000 more deaths than would have occurred at average English mortality rates, a reduction in expectation of life of 12.5 years for each adult in the city. Assuming average production from each adult of 10 shillings a week, this amounted to a loss to the national product of £53,655,550 a year. Even the extra funerals cost £18,000 a year.

Rightly pointing out the relative futility of Liverpool's 27 physicians, 325 surgeons and apothecaries, and 365 chemists and druggists, who could through personal care only alleviate but not prevent sickness, he raged at the pitiful proposals of the wealthy Liverpool Corporation to appoint one medical inspector at a salary of £300 a year, with permission to supplement this with private practice. In contrast to its later defence of private practice in virtually all circumstances, the *Journal* gave full space and implied support to Chadwick's rejection of medical trade as any solution to health problems, quoting him as follows:

> For the more important business of *prevention* . . . it appears that the Corporation propose to appoint one officer only, and to pay very little more than £1 per thousand of the persons whose general health it will be his business to protect . . . My estimate of the service requisite for the initiation of measures of prevention in Liverpool was of three or four officers of health at the least, giving their whole time to the service, at an expense of £2,200 per

> annum . . . But the intended compensation for the inadequate pecuniary provision for the services of one officer that he may take private practice, is entirely destructive of all efficiency . . . Regular private practice not only acts constantly as an inducement to the neglect of regular public duties, but often as a severe penalty for the proper performance of them. In tracing the causes of epidemics, the officer of health must at least occasionally find it in the mismanaged or neglected state of properties owned by his patients, or by persons holding local public office, persons of powerful influence, who sooner or later may exert it to his prejudice . . . Ordinary service must be secured by the ordinary motives to integrity. I do not hesitate to say that the State which lays its foundations in the rare and heroic virtues will be sure to have its superstructure in the basest profligacy and corruption.

He was endorsed by the *Journal*'s editorialist:

> . . . the forgoing remarks, though applied to the individual case before us, are capable of being extended to other localities, and to other official medical duties performed throughout the country for a very inadequate amount of remuneration, for the smallness of which the opportunities afforded for private practice have been held out as an inducement and a compensation. We rejoice to see Mr Chadwick taking so just a view of these transactions . . .

Radical reform versus respectability

Militancy over medical pay for care of the poor was restrained by a countervailing and eventually dominant search for the security and gentlemanly status associated with care for people who could afford fees rather than collective arrangements for prepaid care.[10,11]

For most of the nineteenth century, most skilled medical and surgical procedures were performed in the home, and the *Journal*'s papers were relevant to the everyday practice of most of its readers. Today, the differences between consultant physicians and general practitioners arise from divisions of labour, but for most of the nineteenth century they arose mainly from differences between the social classes they served. Purchasing power determined the time available for consultation, which tended towards hours for the rich, minutes for the poor, and therefore state-of-the-art diagnosis for the one and snap diagnosis for the other.[12]

By the beginning of the twentieth century this search for respectability was dominant, partly because of improved standards of living in the skilled working class, but also because the profession was dividing into GPs and specialists. The emerging and fiercely defended ethical rules of referral removed the consultants from the top end of the GP market,[13] and opened new possibilities for GPs to escape from degrading care of the degraded poor to respectable practice for respectable classes. Teaching hospital consultants, nearly all of them in part-time private practice with wealthy patients, defined the profession in their own image and stamped their views on the BMA and its journal. Though few GPs could practise in that image, they could aspire to it and accept it as their clinical and social goal, and that is exactly what they did for the next eighty years.

The grand old Duke of York: his wars of 1912 and 1948

By the run-up to the First World War, the urban profession was clearly dividing into three main groups: community-based generalists excluded from hospital work; hospital-based consultants losing direct contact with the public; and public health doctors isolated from both. We gained a referral system which gave all but the richest patients to the general practitioner, and all but the smallest hospitals to the specialists. Though this perception by Rosemary Stevens[13] was profoundly true, these essentially rational and cost-effective divisions of labour took another thirty years to complete. To contemporaries this process was obscured by long rearguard actions: by consultants to retain direct access as generalists to the really rich, and by cottage hospital GP surgeons, obstetricians and Harley Street specialoids, to preserve trade in clinical skills they had learned in teaching hospitals, but without a modern hospital base.

These losing battles began in 1911 with the Lloyd George Insurance Bill, and finally ended in 1948 with the NHS. First and last, the BMA and its *Journal* began by accepting principles none could oppose with any hope of public credibility or support, and ended by rejecting them in any feasible legislative form.

Both battles followed the same sequence, inspired by the grand old Duke of York. Up the hill they marched, from rhetorical discussion of reforms in principle to their rejection in practice. Negotiations were broken off, the enemy was accused of planning horrific bureaucratic atrocities, and war was declared, with mass pledges to boycott the service. At the top of the hill they found legislation in place, with massive public support and majorities in parliament. Angry and confused, they first marched, then ran down the hill and into the service. None of those sworn to boycott both Acts actually did so; minor concessions long available were hailed as victories. At regimental reunions thirty years later, both Acts were recalled with affection, recognized as necessary and inevitable, never really opposed by anyone, indeed almost invented by the Duke himself.

The Lloyd George Bill proposed what amounted to nationalization of club and contract practice funded by locally controlled mutual aid societies for care of the industrial working class, creating a new and more comprehensive system of state insurance covering most employed men, but not their families. This promised, and ultimately gave, urban and industrial GPs security and a better income for care of the poor but trapped them in a pattern of industrialized care requiring few recognized clinical skills, from which escape to hospital practice was no longer feasible. Neither Lloyd George nor Bevan offered any serious public investment in primary care, but Bevan did propose planned state investment in hospitals. GPs could therefore be mobilized to oppose the Lloyd George Act in 1912 by consultants who had nothing to gain from it. GPs could still mobilize themselves against that Act's logical successor, the NHS Act in 1948, which extended this pattern of primary care to everyone, and virtually ended fee-earning private general practice, but this time the consultants had slipped off to make their own arrangements.

A spoon-fed race

Both in 1912 and in 1948, doctors and their journal acted in a social and political context impossible to ignore. Across the whole political spectrum, 1912 was a time of upheaval and radicalism. The last decade of the nineteenth century saw the birth of mass socialist parties throughout Europe and the beginnings of independent working-class politics in Britain. Industrial unionism was running through docks, mines and engineering industries in a rising tide of militancy, ended only by the outbreak of world war. Lloyd George tried to regain the workers' vote for the Liberals by bold class legislation, squeezing the spoiled nobility for its cash, and laying foundations for the welfare state. Tory and Liberal imperialists eagerly adopted vulgarized theories of social Darwinism to justify occupation of a quarter of the earth's surface by the British Empire, and most of what remained by other 'less vigorous' white races. Arguments about the Lloyd George Act reflected all these ideas, as well as the bread and butter concerns of GPs. Though the Association tried to express support in principle for the Act while objecting to its terms, inevitably the argument drew energy from wider conflicts.

Sir James Barr,[14] president-elect of the BMA, furiously attacked the Act in terms Margaret Thatcher might recognize. It was, he wrote:

> a long step in the downward path towards socialism. It will tend to destroy individual effort and increase that spirit of dependency which is ever found in degenerate races. This spoon-fed race will look more and more to a paternal government to feed and clothe it, and not require it to work more than a few hours daily. They will be further encouraged to multiply their breed at the expense of the healthy and intellectual members of the community . . . The wage earner is the individual who is best able to take care of himself, and every one who is worthy of his salt does so, and the less unnecessary interference he has with his liberty the better for the State . . . If this Act be allowed to remain on the Statute Book it will set back the hands of the medical clock for at least a quarter of a century, and in future prevent the intellectual youths of the country from entering the medical profession. If the money wasted by the State in all manner of useless schemes for the supposed betterment of the people were employed to encourage the multiplication of the intelligent and vigorous, there might be some chance for the country.

He was duly elected president in 1912, reiterated these views in his inaugural address,[15] and was vigorously supported in a *BMJ* editorial.[16]

Arguments of the same kind resurfaced in 1948. Evelyn Waugh described Britain after the unexpected, and to him incomprehensible, Labour landslide of 1945 as resembling life under enemy occupation. Fifty-eight per cent of professionals had voted Conservative in the election; hostility to the NHS at its birth, from the press as well as from the profession, owed much to this fact. Conversely, 42 per cent of professionals had not voted Conservative, but the real possibility of mobilizing GPs in favour of the Act was lost when the health centres programme, the only planned investment in general practice, was abandoned.

As in 1911, the Association proclaimed support for the principles of the NHS while opposing its terms, but that is not how its more vigorous supporters expressed themselves. Six months before the appointed day, the *Journal* published a speech by Dr Reginald Payne to a special meeting of the Royal College of Surgeons in which he foretold the fate of clinicians under the NHS:[17]

> . . . no patient or doctor will ever feel safe from interference by some ministerial edict or regulation, and no independent institution connected with medicine will feel safe from interference, expropriation, or dissolution. The Minister's spies will be everywhere and suspicion and intrigue will rule.

Ideas of this sort are typical of correspondence in the *Journal* throughout the year preceding the Act. During the first three months of 1948, it published 265 letters on the NHS; 27 (10 per cent) approved or accepted the Act, 35 (13 per cent) wanted compromise, and 203 (77 per cent) opposed the NHS, mostly as final catastrophe. The BMA's leaders, backed by the *Journal*, steadfastly refused negotiations with the Minister, and did all they could to secure an overwhelming vote against participation in the service. They were successful. In an 84 per cent poll, 95 per cent of GPs voted not to participate; but the NHS started on time, and two months later 90 per cent of GPs were working in it.

Commanding heights of the medical economy

Though most consultants probably hated the Labour government as much as any other privileged group, they were also interested in skilled practice, and knew they could not run hospitals from their own pockets. Merit Awards compensated for loss of private practice, which in many cases failed to occur; where it survived, they had their cake and ate it. Their mouths were choked with gold but, more importantly, consultants gained full control of virtually all the machinery of medical production, with state funding, not flag days.

For GPs, the real fight on both occasions was about the survival of 20-minute consultations for a few patients rather than two minutes for everyone, but the leaders of general practice were no longer in the self-critical mood of the nineteenth century. They could not admit the real state of clinical medicine in industrial practice. It is no accident that the Collings Report[18] appeared in *The Lancet*, or that the *BMJ* tried to refute it through the Hadfield Report[19] (though this only confirmed its main conclusions). The situation Collings described, familiar to every industrial GP, could have provided their most powerful argument for an adequately staffed, housed and equipped service; but egged on by their leaders and their *Journal*, the GPs insisted on total autonomy. They were therefore unable to admit the existence of bad work, caused not by personal failings, but by conditions and resources which precluded good work. They scorned public investment, while lacking the will or resources to invest in primary care themselves.

Unable to fight for autonomy with the truth, they used lies which deceived none but themselves. The threat of a salaried service was invented by Charles Hill, Guy Dain and the BMA, not by Aneurin Bevan, who had little faith or interest in general practice. Like most of his contemporaries, he saw the future in terms of hospital specialism, and from the first negotiations with the BMA, readily renounced the Labour Party's 1934 commitment to a full-time salaried service for general practice. To its shame, the *Journal* vigorously propagated that lie, a fact not changed by its penultimate retreat when impending defeat was obvious, and the professional hysteria the *Journal* had helped to create had to be wound down.

John Marks, Stephen Lock and other honest men who, like me, lived through that time, have convinced themselves that neither the BMA nor its *Journal* opposed the birth of the NHS. This belief seems to me to require enormous effort, and serves no useful cause I can understand. Kenneth Clarke is using an essentially accurate folk memory of medical opposition to the birth of the NHS to justify his refusal to listen to us now, when we oppose its death and transfiguration to his new world of internal markets. The answer to this lie is not to contrive a bigger one claiming that doctors have always been right, but freely to admit that we have learned important lessons from the NHS, which have changed the way we see ourselves in relation to society and the state.

You are the jury for this important question, and your evidence sits on the shelf of any library with *BMJ*s for the second half of 1947 and the first half of 1948. Read the editorials and correspondence columns, make your own judgements, and don't let me or anyone else revise history unchallenged. Informed contemporaries, who saw these events from a standpoint very different from mine, took a tougher view of the matter. Lord Platt summed up what later became the consensus and by no means radical view, when he wrote in 1963:[20]

> The methods of the BMA were those of trades unionists, not appropriate to the leadership of a great profession . . . a generation of doctors had been taught to disparage British medicine, to regard the Ministry of Health as its enemy, and to speak of the Health Service in terms of contempt.

The *British Medical Journal* and the new general practice

As Somerville Hastings[21] said, at the birth of the NHS the GPs asked to be left alone so they were left alone, by a government only too pleased to fund a cheap and generally nasty cottage industry, rather than have to provide the network of health centres promised in the 1945 Labour manifesto.

Inclusion of the whole population in a single uniform service without fees, and developments in medical science which expanded the potential for simple and effective treatment outside hospitals, created a framework within which general practice could develop not as a specialoid parody of hospital care, but in its own right. As a mainly patrician concept, this began with the foundation of the Royal College of General Practitioners in 1952, as a defensive move against what was then seen and felt as the degradation of practice easily recognized in the Collings report, which was in many ways the College's founding document.

As plebeian reality and a positive development of the NHS, however, progress in general practice depended on investment of substantial social resources for primary care, which came only in 1967. The GP Charter of 1966 followed an explosion of discontent in a work-force, previously taken for granted, that was recognized at the eleventh hour as essential to the viability of the state. Having lost its GPs and shifted almost entirely to hospital and specialoid care, the United States, the world's richest country, could no longer afford the costs of modern medicine. Our government recognized at last that in the UK we still had GPs, albeit in an increasingly demoralized state. Kenneth Robinson for government, and Jim Cameron for the BMA had the wisdom to see that the only solution was to invest in general practice, in such a way that at least some of the money would be spent on improving patient care, and not simply remain in GPs' pockets as compensation for the unrewarding nature of perfunctory work at high speed over long hours. The BMA and its *Journal* accepted in 1966 what they could and should have fought for with public support in 1948 – serious investment in general practice.

Thoughtful GPs who worked through those times now see the 1966 Charter as the turning point for NHS general practice. It encouraged the first serious programme of health centre building and support for purpose-built practice premises, which ended front-parlour surgeries and the dirty shop on the high street. It encouraged group practice and the employment of secretarial and nursing staff. It created for the first time a serious training programme for new entrants, independent from hospital care and under the control of GP tutors, which in turn provided the chief material base for the Royal College of General Practitioners and its main practical task until it began to run out of steam in the 1980s.

The advances made possible by the Charter were permissive, not mandatory. They made a lot of difference where progress was easiest and least needed, much less difference in areas of urban decay and industrial decline. State investment still depended on individual GP initiative. Innovation by GPs in poor areas still meant a higher workload but lower net income, even under the Charter.[22] However, the Charter remains the best model yet for advance in general practice, and opened a rich new field for the *Journal*.

Over the following two decades, the *British Medical Journal* established itself as the most effective and widely read outlet for an increasing flow of good, mainly descriptive but occasionally experimental literature from general practice. In the 1950s, an unused examination couch loaded with unopened rolls of the *British Medical Journal* was a common feature of industrial practice. Thirty years later that situation had changed. For the first time for almost a century, the *British Medical Journal* could be truly described as useful to and generally used by GPs who cared about the quality of their work.

Privatization of the medical press

The medical press set the scene for the crisis preceding the 1966 Charter, with the usual threats of resignation from the NHS and reversion to private practice, predictably supported by the *BMJ* and opposed by *The Lancet*. This time, however, both stars were upstaged by a new set of downmarket ham actors. These were the new weekly medical news magazines distributed free to GPs and paid for by pharmaceutical advertisers, since known as 'comics', 'freebies', 'trash' and other insulting titles. Starting with *Pulse* in the early 1960s, these provided review articles on clinical topics, free advertising for locums, sale of surplus dogs, cats and unwanted wedding presents, a wide range of interesting medical gossip which peer-reviewed journals were too well-bred to touch, and editorials pandering to the lowest instincts of angry GP entrepreneurs with a style anticipating the worst excesses of contemporary tabloid journalism. As the *BMJ* had done in 1948, they roused the troops to march up the hill, but this time there was a credible forward strategy, so no retreat was necessary. The trash journals won the hearts and minds of a new readership, without paying for them.

This development should be taken seriously by anyone who cares about professional development. Ever since the mid-1960s, these have been the journals most GPs and trainees actually read. In 1988 I found only two out of a group of 30 trainees who gave any subscription journal (the *BMJ* in both cases) as the source of their last clinical reading; all the others recalled one of the trash journals. They said the freebies gave them more of what they actually wanted, more cheaply and easily than any subscription journal. Just as bad currency drives out good, free journals offering instant clinical wisdom and business success threaten the institutional press.

One reason that the *BMJ* offered so few good review articles on commonplace clinical topics of practical value to GPs was the eventual ascendancy in this field of its competitor, the *Practitioner,* founded in 1868. Good GPs counted on and paid for the *Practitioner,* not the *BMJ,* to update them once a month on significant clinical advances in everyday practice; a readable, reliable, conservative and didactic journal, which lost most of its circulation and all of its dignity as soon as the freebies were able to offer the same material vulgarized for painless reading at zero cost. In large parts of the world, virtually all of South and Central America for example, general subscription journals have virtually ceased to exist. In Italy a free medical newspaper appears three times a week, and there is no longer any independent general medical journal.

Peer-reviewed journals are national and international institutions, their economics a mystery. To have a paper accepted, even a letter, is an honour, and there is therefore no question of paying for it. The trash press is both a privatization and a popularization of medical journalism, very much on the tabloid model. It operates frankly for profit and to entertain. Anything goes, so long as it sells, and pleases the advertisers. It will endorse both entrepreneurial practice and the habit of prescribing at least something for everything, whether or not these policies assist the accurate delivery of medical science to those who need it. To the extent that subscription journals were too pompous and defensive to see the need for news that mirrored more faithfully what really goes on in practice, and the practical needs of GPs, they had only themselves to blame.

A free journal is like a free lunch; someone is paying, and for a purpose. *The Lancet* is lost in its laboratory somewhere in mid-Atlantic, having abandoned its GP readers. The *BMJ* is now probably the best general medical journal in the world, but cannot compete on equal terms; it costs money, and GPs have learned to expect everything free, from their postgraduate education to their videotapes. The real cost is to the common people, both ways: through their taxes for the NHS, which pay for the prescribed drugs promoted by the advertisers who pay the costs of producing trash journals; and through the care they receive from GPs whose brains are washed once a week in the interests of the pharmaceutical industry. This distorted and socially counterproductive economy can and should be rectified by legislative change.

The *British Medical Journal* in defence of society and the National Health Service

By the late 1970s, British GPs and the *BMJ* had learned to love the National Health Service. Pursuit of better clinical practice unimpeded by fees, or by any consideration other than the needs of patients and our present state of knowledge, was a wonderful and for the first time credible state, actually existing for some clinicians and conceivable for all. Consensus had been achieved on the social arrangements for delivery of medical care, and it seemed only a matter of time and hard work to continue a medical progress in which professional knowledge rather than money would be the rate-limiting factor.

This belief was wrong on two counts. First, what appeared to be a permanent consensus on the welfare state proved to be ephemeral. There was no guarantee of permanent funding for anything, however admirable or socially necessary, which did not pay its own way through profit. Half a century of progress in social legislation began to unravel, and no end is in sight. If medical care returns to the market, state medical services will slide back a century, becoming again a squalid last resort for paupers, from which all doctors who can, will escape. In medicine as throughout society, social retreat, concealed by technical advance, will be hailed as progress.

Second, less obviously, but in the long run more importantly, effective application of medical science to real people depends not only on what doctors know and understand, but also on active and creative participation by patients. The traditional aims of medicine assumed that if all providers knew and all consumers obeyed, better health would follow. This strategy is fundamentally false. We cannot relate effectively to society as producers of care consumed passively by our populations, whether as a marketed commodity or a public service. Progress depends on recognizing that production of better health can come only from the combined work of two sets of experts,[12,23] health workers who understand human biology, and patients and their families who understand the personal circumstances within which their problems arise and must be solved.

Understanding of this second problem is a precondition for overcoming the first. Without something better than the obsolete provider–consumer model, there is no alternative to the market, and appeals to conscience or sentimentality are as ineffective today as they were in the nineteenth century. Over the past decade the *Journal* has thundered, better than ever before, over social evils such as unemployment and our barbaric prison service, and against the imposition of a market economy in the NHS, but it has scarcely begun to elaborate an alternative.

My inevitably selective reading of the *BMJ* over the past 150 years leads to a hopeful conclusion. For the first 50 years or so we were active and caring members of the human race, and shared its insecurity. For about the next 80 years, we thought we were the fittest, had survived, and could escape the common fate. For the last 20 years, slowly and hesitatingly at first, now more confidently, we are rediscovering a more modest but much more effective place in a world which, in these terribly dangerous times, will need our help to survive. We should honour our *Journal* for helping to develop the courage and imagination we shall need for that task.

Acknowledgements

I am grateful to the Medical Research Council for giving me time to prepare this paper, to the librarians at the British Medical Association's Nuffield Library, and to Dr Irvine Loudon for advice.

Notes

1. J. Brotherston, 'Memorandum of evidence of the BMA' in G. McLachlan and T. McKeown (eds) *Medical History and Medical Care*, London: Oxford University Press, 1971.

2. Committee of Poor Law Medical Convention, on Poor Law medical relief, *Provincial Medical and Surgical Journal* 1848; 8: 389–90.

3. I. Loudon, *Medical Care and the General Practitioner 1750–1850*, Oxford: Clarendon Press, 1986.

4. Editorial. 'Report on a meeting of Union Medical Officers', *Provincial Medical and Surgical Journal* 1847; 7: 574–5.

5. Editorial. 'Ill-treatment of a Union Medical Officer', *Provincial Medical and Surgical Journal* 1848; 8: 68–9.

6. 'Medical intelligence. Mortality of medical practitioners in Ireland from fever', *Provincial Medical and Surgical Journal* 1848; 8: 83.

7. Editorial. 'Medical regulations of Friendly Societies', *Provincial Medical and Surgical Journal* 1848; 8: 40–1.

8. *The Battle of the Clubs.* Reprint of the reports of the special commissioner of *The Lancet* appointed to enquire into the Medical Aid Societies, London: Lancet, 1896.

9. Editorial. 'Health of towns: medical inspectors', *Provincial Medical and Surgical Journal* 1847; 7: 70–2.

10. N. Parry and J. Parry, *The Rise of the Medical Profession*, London: Croom Helm, 1976.

11. M.J. Peterson, *The Medical Profession in Mid-Victorian London*, Los Angeles and London: University of California Press, 1978.

12. J.T. Hart, *A New Kind of Doctor*, London: Merlin Press, 1988.

13. R. Stevens, *Medical Practice in Modern England: The Impact of Specialization and State Medicine*, New Haven and London: Yale University Press, 1966.

14. J. Barr, 'Some reasons why the public should oppose the Insurance Act', *British Medical Journal* 1911; ii: 1713–15.

15. J. Barr, 'What are we? What are we doing here? Whence do we come and whither do we go?' *British Medical Journal* 1912; ii: 157–62.

16. Editorial. 'The racial responsibility of medicine', *British Medical Journal* 1912; ii: 186–7.

17. Quoted in M. Foot, *Aneurin Bevan: A Biography. Volume II, 1945–1960*, London: Davis Poynter, 1973, p. 165.

18. J.S. Collings, 'General practice in England today', *Lancet* 1950; i: 555–85.

19. S.J. Hadfield, 'A field survey of general practice', *British Medical Journal* 1953; 2: 683–706.

20. R. Platt, *Doctor and Patient: Ethics, Morale, Government*, London: Nuffield Provincial Hospitals Trust, 1963.

21. S. Hastings, 'General practitioners in the National Health Service', *Lancet* 1950; i: 882.

22. N. Bosanquet and B. Leese, 'Family doctors and innovation in general practice', *British Medical Journal* 1988; 296: 1576–80.

23. D. Tuckett, M. Boulton, C. Olson and A. Williams, *Meetings Between Experts: An Approach to Sharing Ideas in Medical Consultations*, London: Tavistock Publications, 1985.

13

The *British Medical Journal* and the twentieth-century consultant

Christopher C. Booth

At the beginning of this century there were relatively few physicians or surgeons who worked as consultants to hospitals and were successful in private practice in their chosen specialty. When consulted, they often had little to offer. For all that, they had an inordinate influence on the affairs of their profession. Those who were not Fellows of either of the two influential and powerful Royal Colleges of Physicians or Surgeons counted for little in the medical hierarchy, being, like Chesterfield's women, neither consulted about nor trusted with serious matters. Privileged consultants who enjoyed an attachment to a prestigious teaching hospital in London reigned supreme, and women themselves occupied the lowly position of playthings to which the Earl of Chesterfield had consigned them a century and a half earlier.

There has been no period of human history to compare with the half-century since 1900 during which so many advances in science and technology have revolutionized the practice of medicine. In the words of Sir Henry Dale, written in 1950, 'our successors . . . are likely to recognise the first half of the 20th century as the period in which civilisation first began to feel, for good or ill, the full impact of progress in the natural sciences'.[1] By 1900 radiology, following Roentgen's discovery of X-rays in 1895, was beginning to be exploited and thyroid treatment had been introduced by Murray for the treatment of cretinism or myxoedema – his original paper having been published in the *British Medical Journal* in 1891. Diphtheria antitoxin was in routine use and Almroth Wright's typhoid vaccine was being tried out in the South African War. Tetanus antitoxin and different forms of active immunization were to follow, particularly in the prevention and treatment of diphtheria. The later identification of the sulphonamides and arsenicals led to successful chemotherapy. Antimalarials were developed and Alexander Fleming's discovery of penicillin was followed by its isolation and purification by Florey and Chain, an event which led to the introduction of a whole range of antibiotics effective against both aerobic and anaerobic infections.

The discovery of insulin and other hormones made a huge impact on medical practice during this era as did the recognition of the vitamins as important in the prevention of certain types of nutritional deficiency disease. Perhaps the most impressive of these – to the clinical consultant – was the discovery by the future Nobel laureates Minot and Murphy that pernicious anaemia could be treated with a liver diet. Others showed that the disorder is due to a deficiency of vitamin B12 and that this deficiency, unlike other nutritional deficiency diseases which are due to dietary inadequacy, is caused by a failure of absorption of the vitamin as a result of the lack of an intrinsic factor secreted by the stomach. And that, as we now know, is due to an autoimmune gastritis.

So much more has been discovered – agents which can relieve pain, anaesthetic substances which are safe to use, drugs to lower blood pressure, and the all-important identification of the structure of DNA with all the advances in molecular biology which have followed. At the same time, imaging techniques have made the human body virtually transparent and there is no part of it that the surgeon does not now dare to invade.

Nor should one forget the importance of modern statistics and epidemiology and the pioneering work of Doll and Bradford Hill on cancer of the lung.[2] The controlled clinical trial is also a feature of this century and, as Michael Shepherd has shown, subjects such as psychiatry have come to take their proper place in clinical research. At the same time, with the development of modern methods of communication and travel, medicine has become increasingly internationalized. The eradication of smallpox through the efforts of the World Health Organisation and the virtual conquest of cholera by multidisciplinary and multinational teams are perhaps the two greatest achievements of international cooperation.

Many of these developments have been associated with advances in technology. Antisepsis, antibiotics, anaesthesia, blood transfusion, fluid replacement and heart-lung machines have made modern cardiac surgery possible. We can now transplant the heart, liver and kidney, to say nothing of pancreatic islets. Tiny babies born prematurely may now survive in specialized intensive care units. But all these new technologies require trained personnel if survival is to be assured after the physician or surgeon has doffed his gown and gone home.

The expansion of the work-force involved in health care has been a major development during the twentieth century. As specialties have developed in response to medical advances, a vast new range of consultant staff has become necessary, all demanding the same status and privileges as those who have gone before, so that new royal colleges, whose presidents have been invariably rewarded by recognition in the honours systems so beloved of the British, have become inevitable. At the same time, the function of the clinical consultant has changed from that of one who looked into his hospital, giving his opinion, perhaps doing some teaching, operating if he was a surgeon, to one who may be the leader of a team using significant resources which may compete with other equally significant demands on the public purse. He has in addition demanded support by an increasing army of junior medical staff for whose postgraduate education he has become responsible.

The increase in medical manpower has involved a wide range of disciplines.[3] As an example, there were in 1900 no more than 305 Fellows of the Royal College of Physicians of London. By 1940 there were 619 and now the figure has risen to 5,736. Members of the College, predominantly trainees, have increased from 452 in 1900 to 17,616 today. At the same time there has been a great increase in the number of individuals working in disciplines ancillary to medicine. In the United States, for example, there were estimated to be about 345,000 persons working in health care at the beginning of this century and of these one in three was a physician, using the word in the American sense of practitioner. By 1976, the United States health work-force had grown to about 5.1 million and only one in thirteen of these was a physician. The allied health occupations (and these figures exclude nursing and nursing auxiliaries) contained 155 recognized specialties in 1976 – physiotherapists, radiographic technicians, laboratory assistants and so on. In Britain too there have been similar developments so that the consultant of the twentieth century has come to be simply one among a group of health workers, albeit a leading member, serving the community in which he lives, rather than being the totally independent professional that he was at the beginning of the century, a time when he enjoyed great individual kudos and prestige. It is a change of status that has not been relished by older and more paternalist consultants, many of whom have not felt entirely easy with the new era of openness and explanation that a more informed public opinion has imposed upon them. The response of professional bodies such as the Royal Colleges has been to encourage audit and accountability. But as Rudolph Klein has so cogently put it, it would all be very well if it were not that the profession's current more responsible attitude didn't have a ring of death-bed repentance about it.

The changes in the practice of medicine that have so radically altered the life of the twentieth-century consultant have occurred equally in other western nations, notably the United States. Yet there have been other developments, specific to Britain, that have been of equal if not greater importance in this country. The introduction of the National Health Service in 1948 dramatically changed the consultant in the prestigious voluntary hospital from an unpaid individual who earned his living in private practice and gave his services without remuneration to a salaried servant of the emerging health service. As the service developed through the years, consultant services were increasingly built up on a regional basis so that the major cities, such as London and Edinburgh, Glasgow, Manchester and so on, no longer remained the medical Meccas that they had traditionally been and the provincial consultant gradually achieved a status of equality with his metropolitan counterpart. The National Health Service had a further important influence on consultants. If one excludes distinction awards, the remuneration of consultants in the Health Service was similar in all specialties so that the psychiatrist, geriatrician and neurosurgeon were all paid at equal rates, a great encouragement to the development of what were undoubtedly 'cinderella' specialties, for example geriatric medicine or mental handicap.

The modern university-based medical school has also been a feature of this century, particularly in England, where full-time professorships in the clinical subjects did not exist until after the ending of the First World War. At the same time, research became an increasing concern for those practising as consultants in the medical schools. The foundation of the Medical

Research Council in its present form dates from 1920 and since that time there has been increasing pressure for clinical research workers to be awarded honorary consultant contracts, particularly – though not exclusively – in the teaching hospitals. At the same time, charitable foundations such as the Imperial Cancer Research Fund began to have an important supplementary role to that of the government in the support of research, as the Wellcome Trust does today.

These changes that have so profoundly affected the lives of consultants have been faithfully reflected in the pages of the *British Medical Journal* through the century, as can be seen by examining issues of the *Journal* decade by decade. In the first issue for the year 1900, for example, there was 'A clinical lecture on minor epilepsy' by Sir William Gowers, the *Journal* providing then, as it was to do for many years, ample space for the expression of their unrefereed views by the medical grandees of the day. There were also extensive reports of the meetings of medical societies and that first issue of 1900 carried, a reflection of Britain's then Imperial position, the record of the 'medical and surgical practice in the hospitals and asylums of the British Empire'. From Barbados there was an account of the amputation of a leg grossly deformed by elephantiasis. The leg, the *Journal* solemnly declared, was sent to the Secretary of State for the Colonies – for onward transmission to the School for Tropical Medicine in Greenwich. The war in South Africa was reported in a paper from Cape Town. Yet in terms of the status of consultants at that time there can have been nothing so revealing as the obituary of Sir James Paget who had died only a day or two before the opening of the new century. The obituary notice occupied five and a half pages of double column. Paget was buried in Westminster Abbey and one of the pallbearers was Lord Lister.

A decade later, after the customary addresses by distinguished consultants on subjects such as ureteral calculi and 'the rational puerperium', the *Journal*, saluting the new decade, recorded that 'Welcome ever smiles, and farewell goes out sighing'. The particular reason for sighing in that year has an almost contemporary ring, since 1909 had been a bad year for trade and the medical profession had not escaped the general depression. It was by no means unique to that issue that the leader writer expressed the hope that the New Year would 'bring to the country increased prosperity . . . in which the medical profession may reasonably expect to share . . .'.

In 1920, after the horror and bloodshed of Flanders, the major article of the first issue of the decade was an oration by Sir Anthony Bowlby on gunshot wounds of the femur – there had been many. The issue also carried the obituary of Sir William Osler who had died on 29 December 1919. At three and a half pages, two less than for Paget, it was a formidable tribute to a great man of medicine. The *Journal* has always faithfully recorded the ribbons, bangles and stars accorded to medical men, most of them consultants. That same issue carried the news of Sir Bertrand Dawson's elevation to a hereditary peerage.

In January 1930, the *Journal* gave extensive coverage to the Edinburgh physician Edwin Bramwell for an address on some aspects of pain. There was also a reflection of the clinical problems of yesteryear, an article on syphilitic appendicitis. During those decades, no consultant, particularly if he worked in a prestigious London teaching hospital, could complain that the *BMJ* did not accord him enough opportunity to share his thoughts with lesser mortals. The first issue of 1940, published during that quiet period of the phoney war, contained the Harveian Oration given at the Royal College of Physicians by R.A. Young of the Middlesex and Brompton Hospitals on 'The pulmonary circulation before and after Harvey'. Who remembers him, or that, now? By this time sulphonamides were available and were being tried in bacterial endocarditis. And the BMA was setting up a committee to report on nutrition in wartime.

But one of the most remarkable issues of the *Journal*, a goldmine for the historian, was the first for the year 1950. Saluting fifty years of medicine, the initial article was a *tour de force* by Sir Henry Dale on the subject of 'Advances in medical therapeutics'. The remaining articles were by the leading medical men of the day – Sir Geoffrey Jefferson, R.W. Johnstone, Sir Henry (later Lord) Cohen, Sir Lionel Whitby, Sir John Boyd, Cochrane Shanks and Sir Arthur MacNalty. The distinguished medical historian Charles Singer was also recruited, contributing an admirable piece on medicine between 1850 and 1900. The entire issue was a panegyric to the remarkable advances in medicine that had occurred by mid-century. By then the National Health Service had been established and subsequent issues of the *Journal* were increasingly to reflect the concerns of the profession and of consultants during the development of the service.

Ten years later, in the first issue for 1960, the *Journal* again published a lengthy account of a Lumleian lecture at the Royal College of Physicians – 'Clinical and metabolic studies in thyroid disease' by E.J. Wayne, professor of medicine in the University of Glasgow. Antibiotic resistance was now an important topic and the relationship between ABO blood groups and secretor status was being reported by C.A. Clarke and his colleagues in Liverpool. There were also contributions on dietary methods for lowering plasma lipids, a subject that has obstinately refused to go away. The obituary notices of the great and the good had now shrunk to as little as two and a half columns at most.

By 1970, there had been a pronounced change in the *Journal* both in format and in style. The *Journal* now began with its leading articles and there was to be a striking reduction in the publication of the formal lecture by some distinguished consultant. In that issue, however, the vexed question of 'Epidemic malaise', which had appeared as Royal Free Disease in 1955, was reconsidered, as it was to be repeatedly in subsequent years. There was now an increasing concern with the publication of properly conducted clinical trials.

1980 witnessed the early years of the Thatcher era. The first leading article bewailed 'The flight from science'. Vancouver style was introduced. There was a student writing about his elective and 'Scrutator' recorded the moving of the second reading of a new Health Service Bill by the then Secretary of State, Patrick Jenkin, a promise of things to come.

By 1990, the *Journal*'s more positive approach to medicine in the modern era, and its increasing readability, were engagingly apparent. On the scientific side there was an article on colour Doppler flow mapping. There were comments on the MRC's annual report and a guide to GP budgets under the government's new proposals for the National Health Service. The *Journal* had now ventured into quality book publishing and this was reflected by its recommendation of the Keynes Press reprint of Frank Danby's work *Dr Phillips: a Maida Vale idyll*, which dealt with rumoured events, involving wife murder, in the life of that remarkable former editor of the *BMJ*, Ernest Hart.

It has to be admitted that through the years there has not been unanimous enthusiasm for the *BMJ* amongst consultants.

The physician Richard Asher, that brilliant depressive, was expressing a general view when he published an article in the *Journal* in 1958 attacking medical journals for being so dull.[4] Whilst he was writing in general terms, it was clear from his critique of wrappings and covers which were drab and difficult to remove that many of his strictures were directed at the *BMJ*. He was concerned about unattractive titles to papers, bewailed the lack of colour, deplored the amount of junk that got published and was critical of presentation and style. Above all he castigated dullness. Yet one has to accept that not everything is interesting to everyone and it is more than probable that if Asher, whose lively mind required constant stimulation, were to have read Watson and Crick's paper on the double helix, he might well have found that dull.

It was perhaps inevitable that consultants might be critical of the developments that changed medical education during this century, and that their views would be expressed in the columns of the *BMJ*. At the beginning of the century, there were no academic departments in clinical subjects in the medical schools in London, where the majority of medical students learnt their craft. Teaching was entirely in the hands of the consultants to the voluntary hospitals. The aspiring medical student often first took a degree in pre-clinical subjects at Oxford or Cambridge and would return at the end of his clinical training in London to take a clinical degree at his *alma mater*, which examined him without taking any responsibility for his clinical education. The system was popular with the London consultants since it was they, returning to dinner and port in their old colleges, who did the examining. Less favoured students who studied in London often took the qualifying examinations set by the Royal Colleges of Physicians and Surgeons, an important source of finance to them.

The Haldane Report on University Education in London, whose findings were published in the *BMJ* in April 1913, strongly recommended that academic professorial units should be established in the London medical schools.[5] The recommendation followed the pattern set by the German medical schools which had been so effective during the nineteenth century and so influential in the United States. The German model had been enthusiastically endorsed by Abraham Flexner in his own seminal report on American medical education in 1910 and Flexner had been an important witness to the

Haldane Commission. Sir William Osler, who did so much for British medicine during his tenure of the Regius Chair in Oxford, was an equally important voice, expressing the unequivocal view that what was needed in Britain was an active invasion of the hospitals by the universities. In the final report, Haldane stated unhesitatingly that full-time professors in the clinical subjects, with their own laboratories and assistants, should be appointed in the London schools. The report and its recommendations were strongly supported in the pages of the *BMJ* by the distinguished University College physiologist, Professor E.H. Starling.[6]

There were, however, immediate reactions from the London consultants. Some expressed regret that there was not included among the Commission a medical man, preferably a London graduate, who would have been acquainted with the conditions of medical education in London. Starling rejected this argument, pointing out that no other practical subject, for example engineering, had been represented. But many consultants remained vehemently opposed to any change in the *status quo* in London. Their views were set out in no uncertain terms in the *BMJ* by E. Graham Little, dean of the medical school at St Mary's Hospital, a fierce antagonist to national health schemes and to socialism in all its forms and an individual who was no stranger to controversy. He adhered, as did many others, to the Oxbridge system of medical education and wrote that surely most persons would accord to the opinion of the great universities of Oxford and Cambridge as to what constituted teaching of university rank. As to research and the teaching of medicine in Germany, he wrote that doctors from Britain were 'sometimes shocked in Germany by what appears to the English-trained man as callous handling of the sick'.[7] In later years, it was to be for similar reasons that Little's conservative consultant successors in the London schools expressed their serious reservations when invasive techniques such as cardiac catheterization and liver biopsy were introduced at that then radical institution, the Postgraduate Medical School at Hammersmith.

The battle between full-time academics and part-time consultants over who controlled medical education in London was to rumble on for a full half-century. The Haldane proposals were taken up after the First World War when St Bartholomew's Hospital, to its eternal credit, appointed Archibald Garrod as its first full-time professor of medicine. He never took up his post for he was selected to be Osler's successor as the Regius Professor in Oxford a short time afterwards. Soon, however, academic departments were established at St Bartholomew's, University College Hospital, St Mary's and St Thomas'. By 1944, when the Goodenough Report on medical education was published, the move towards academically controlled medical schools had made reasonable headway and it now received enthusiastic support. The report was summarized in the *BMJ*[8] which emphasized the urgent need for the medical schools to begin as soon as possible to make more junior teaching and research appointments. There was a further recommendation that was to have major repercussions for the traditional London schools, which with the exception of the Royal Free Hospital, were predominantly male-dominated at that time. They were to become coeducational. From then on women, who until then had occupied the position of Dr Johnson's lady preacher in the medical profession, increasingly joined the ranks of consultants.

The *Journal* has retained a continuing interest in the affairs of the nation's medical schools, in their teachers and in their research. Welcoming the report of a further Royal Commission on Medical Education chaired by Lord Todd in 1968, the *Journal* pointed to the two underlying themes of that report. 'The first,' explained an anonymous leader writer, 'is that the undergraduate course is to provide not a finished doctor but a person who can become one with further training. The second is that medical education should continue throughout professional life.' The *Journal* was, however, uncertain whether the report might simply be pigeon-holed, its origin, under Mr Harold Wilson, casting 'a shadow over its destiny'.[9]

Consultants, professors and other medical teachers have good reason to be thankful to the *BMJ* for its encouragement of research through the years. In 1920, when the original Medical Research Committee, founded in 1913, became the Medical Research Council, the *Journal* recorded its support for the proposed reorganization and welcomed the maintenance of close links with the universities.[10] The *Journal* was later to give its strong endorsement to Sir Thomas Lewis's views in his campaign within the MRC for support for clinical research. In 1930, Lewis set out to answer the question 'Is there a science of experimental medicine?' posed in the annual report of the Medical Research Council by its then secretary, Sir Walter

Fletcher. In a long article in the *BMJ* Lewis asserted that 'there is indeed a fertile science that deals primarily with patients and this must be encouraged to a more vigorous growth'.[11] He argued strongly for the creation and training of a group of workers who would devote their lives primarily to research, making disease as it occurred in man the centre point of their studies. He believed that clinical science had reached a stage where it should develop its own training ground for new recruits and that it should also achieve independence and freedom. Lewis must have been delighted with the *Journal*'s response. In a leading article, the *BMJ* gave enthusiastic support, concluding: 'The report of the Medical Research Council and Sir Thomas Lewis' clear analysis should go far to convince those who have at heart the progress of medicine in Britain that some posts must be created for research physicians'.[12]

Yet if the *BMJ*'s relationships with teachers and research workers are important in any assessment of its contacts with the twentieth-century consultant, it is in its dialogue with the royal colleges and faculties that represent the consultant hierarchy that the *BMJ*'s views may best be discerned. At the beginning of the century, there were only two royal colleges – the venerable, ancient and dignified Royal College of Physicians, founded in 1518, and the Royal College of Surgeons, whose royal charter had been granted in the nineteenth century. Only one further college emerged before the Second World War, the Royal College of Obstetricians and Gynaecologists which began in 1929. The two other royal colleges had attempted to strangle the new college at birth, fearing that they would lose their monopoly on qualifying examinations, an important source of revenue. The Royal College of Physicians in particular has an unequalled record in attempting to stifle potential competitors. In 1812 it had successfully intervened with the authorities to prevent the newly founded Medical and Chirurgical Society, later the Royal Society of Medicine, from obtaining a royal charter,[13] although it was unable to sustain its position during the reign of William IV. In 1929, however, the *BMJ* was enthusiastic about the proposal to create a third college. 'We offer a cordial welcome to the British College of Obstetricians and Gynaecologists,' wrote their leader writer. 'Our hope,' it went on, 'that harmony will be reached and conflicting views will be adjusted is based on the faith that everyone concerned is animated by the single ideal of raising as high as possible the level of medicine practised in all its branches.'[14]

The Royal College of General Practitioners, whose emergence was also opposed by the Royal College of Physicians, not unnaturally received warm encouragement from the *BMJ* when it was set up in 1952. The *Journal* commended the moving spirits, commenting: 'Those who care for the welfare of medicine will thank them for their expertise and foresight and urge them forward along the path they have courageously taken'.[15]

The foundation of the Royal College of Pathologists was also given strong support by the *BMJ*. In 1962 the *Journal* had pointed to the crisis in esteem that had arisen among pathologists.[16] They were fearful of becoming mere drudges, purveyors of reports. It was also clear that as a postgraduate qualification the membership of the Royal College of Physicians was totally inappropriate and the MD degree was notoriously variable throughout the country. Nevertheless, historians may note that, as far as bacteriology is concerned, Robert Koch with his platinum loop would not feel out of place in a modern laboratory, nor would Virchow be at all surprised by what he would find in the average histopathology laboratory.

The enormous expansion in the number of royal colleges and faculties since the Second World War has been a reflection of the expansion of specialties and their demand for status within the political world of the National Health Service. Colleges have access to the power structure of the Health Service through their membership of the Joint Consultants Committee. There are now colleges of radiologists, anaesthetists, psychiatrists, ophthalmologists, pathologists and so on, and we are facing the prospect of new colleges of paediatricians and dentists. Ancient foundations such as the Royal College of Physicians have therefore found their power base increasingly diluted by other colleges, a situation that has not yet been entirely accepted by their long-serving and conservative officers, whose terms of office have on occasion lasted until death.

The Royal College of Physicians, once described as an institution where slippered medical cardinals discuss preferment, is the only one of the profession's élitist organizations with which the *BMJ* has had a serious altercation. In April 1956, the then editor, Dr Hugh Clegg, wrote an anonymous leading article entitled 'The gold-headed cane'.[17] The piece was an attack upon the president of the Royal College of Physicians, Sir Russell Brain, for standing for office for the seventh successive year. Clegg also criticized the College for failing to come to terms with the emerging world of medicine in a modern welfare state, specifically with the newly established National Health Service, for concerning itself too much with haggling over terms and conditions of service to hospital consultants, for failing to develop postgraduate educational activities (as the Royal College of Surgeons had done) and for their isolation from other bodies such as the BMA and the GMC on questions involving medical education.

Not unnaturally Brain accepted none of these criticisms.[18] Although in retrospect it can be seen that there was a great deal to justify Clegg's censuring of the Royal College and its distinguished president, the BMA establishment of the day rallied to Brain's support. It was only with difficulty that Clegg's editorial freedom was assured. Yet it is now clear that Clegg was entirely right, as illustrated by the College's attitude to the hazards of nicotine. That same year the president was asked by Dr F. Avery Jones (later Sir Francis) to produce a report on the evils of smoking.[19] Brain, a reserved man known for his formidable silences, replied that everyone knew all about the dangers of smoking and went on:

> If we go beyond facts to the question of the giving of advice to the public as to what action they should take in the light of the facts, I doubt very much whether that should be a function of the College.[20]

It was not until a new president, Professor Robert Platt of Manchester, was elected that anything changed. Platt was the first academic to be elected president. He was also a provincial whose election breached, as the *BMJ* put it, 'a London monopoly on one of the high offices of the world of medicine'.[21] It was under Platt's presidency that the College decided to reverse Brain's decision and produce its major contribution to medicine this century – the smoking report.

Looking back to all that has happened over the years of the twentieth century, one of the most significant developments has been the undoubted erosion of the position of the consultant in society, as well as within the profession itself. Yet the downhearted should recognize that this is not something that has happened uniquely to hospital consultants. When, after the death of that great thespian, Lord Olivier, the younger actor Albert Finney was asked whether Olivier's mantle would not now fall upon him, he replied firmly: 'No – there are no Kings and Emperors any more. Now it is a democracy'.

Notes

1. H. Dale, 'Advances in medical therapeutics', *Br Med J* 1950; 1: 1–7.
2. R. Doll and A.B. Hill, 'Lung cancer and other causes of death in relation to smoking', *Br Med J* 1956; 2: 1071–81.
3. C.C. Booth, 'Technology and medicine', *Proc Roy Soc London* (Series B) 1985; 224: 267–85.
4. R. Asher, 'Why are medical journals so dull?' *Br Med J* 1958; 2: 356.
5. Royal Commission on University Education in London. *Report.* London: HMSO, 1910–1913 (Chairman Viscount Haldane).
6. E.H. Starling, 'The report of the Royal Commission in reference to medical teaching in London', *Br Med J* 1913; 1: 1063–5 and 1168–70.
7. E.G. Little, A criticism of Professor Starling's first article [Letter to the Editor]. *Br Med J* 1913; 1: 1170–72.
8. *Report of Interdepartmental Committee on Medical Schools.* (Chairman Sir William Goodenough). London: HMSO, 1944.
9. Anonymous. New look in medicine [Editorial]. *Br Med J* 1968; 2: 65–6.
10. Anonymous. The new Council of Medical Research [Editorial]. *Br Med J* 1920; 1: 510–11.
11. T. Lewis, 'Research in medicine: its position and its needs', *Br Med J* 1930; 1: 479–83.
12. Anonymous. Research physicians [Editorial]. *Br Med J* 1930; 503–4.
13. M. Davidson, *The Royal Society of Medicine.* London: Royal Society of Medicine, 1955: 22.
14. Anonymous. British College of Obstetricians and Gynaecologists [Editorial]. *Br Med J* 1929; 1: 462.
15. Anonymous. The College of General Practitioners [Editorial]. *Br Med J* 1952; 2: 1344–5.
16. Anonymous. College of Pathologists [Editorial]. *Br Med J* 1962: 1: 1258–9.
17. Anonymous. The Gold-headed Cane [Editorial]. *Br Med J* 1956; 1: 791–3.
18. W.R. Brain, The Gold-headed Cane [Letter to the Editor]. *Br Med J* 1956; 1: 918–19.

19. F. Avery Jones, Typescript autograph letter to Sir Russell Brain, 15 November 1956. Brain papers, Royal College of Physicians of London.

20. W.R. Brain, Copy of typescript letter to Dr F. Avery Jones, 13 December 1956. Brain papers, Royal College of Physicians of London.

21. Anonymous. President of the Royal College of Physicians [Editorial]. *Br Med J* 1957; 1: 1000.

Index